By Darakhshan T.S.

Daily Doses of Health

66 Days of Little Reminders to Live Your Best Life

Hello! Readers....

THIS BOOK ISN'T ABOUT RIGID ROUTINES OR SACRIFICES—IT'S ABOUT EMBRACING SIMPLE, JOYFUL MOMENTS THAT MAKE YOU FEEL YOUR BEST.

EACH DAY, YOU'LL FIND SMALL REMINDERS TO SLOW DOWN, BREATHE, AND MAKE CHOICES THAT ALIGN WITH YOUR WELL-BEING. FROM MINDFUL EATING TO RESTFUL SLEEP, AND JOYFUL MOVEMENT TO MOMENTS OF CALM, THESE DAILY DOSES ARE DESIGNED TO FIT EASILY INTO YOUR LIFE.

READY TO START? DIVE IN AND DISCOVER HOW JUST A FEW MINUTES EACH DAY CAN HELP YOU FEEL HEALTHIER, HAPPIER, AND MORE LIKE YOUR BEST SELF.

Why 66 days?

RESEARCH BY DR. PHILLIPPA LALLY AT UNIVERSITY COLLEGE LONDON FOUND THAT, ON AVERAGE, IT TAKES 66 DAYS FOR A NEW BEHAVIOR TO BECOME AUTOMATIC. REPEATING AN ACTION CONSISTENTLY OVER THIS PERIOD HELPS FORM NEURAL PATHWAYS IN THE BRAIN, MAKING THE BEHAVIOR FEEL NATURAL AND REDUCING MENTAL EFFORT. THIS TIMEFRAME IS SCIENTIFICALLY PROVEN TO HELP TURN HEALTHY ACTIONS INTO LASTING HABITS, SETTING THE FOUNDATION FOR LONG-TERM WELL-BEING.

Here's to a life that feels as good as it looks!

Mindful Beginnings

1

Setting the Tone for Health

HEALTH ISN'T ABOUT PERFECTION; IT'S ABOUT PROGRESS. ONE SMALL CHANGE TODAY CAN MAKE A BIG DIFFERENCE TOMORROW.

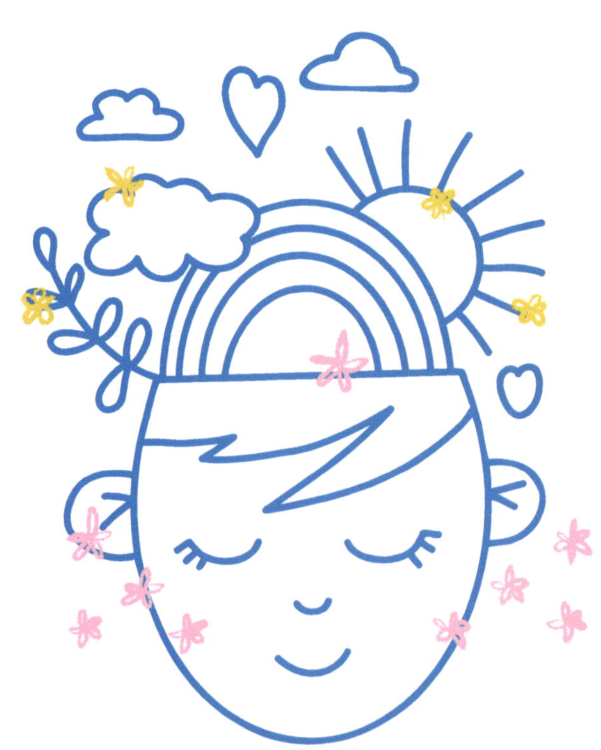

Day 2

PAUSE. BREATHE DEEPLY. IN THIS MOMENT, YOU'RE EXACTLY WHERE YOU NEED TO BE ON YOUR JOURNEY.

Day 3

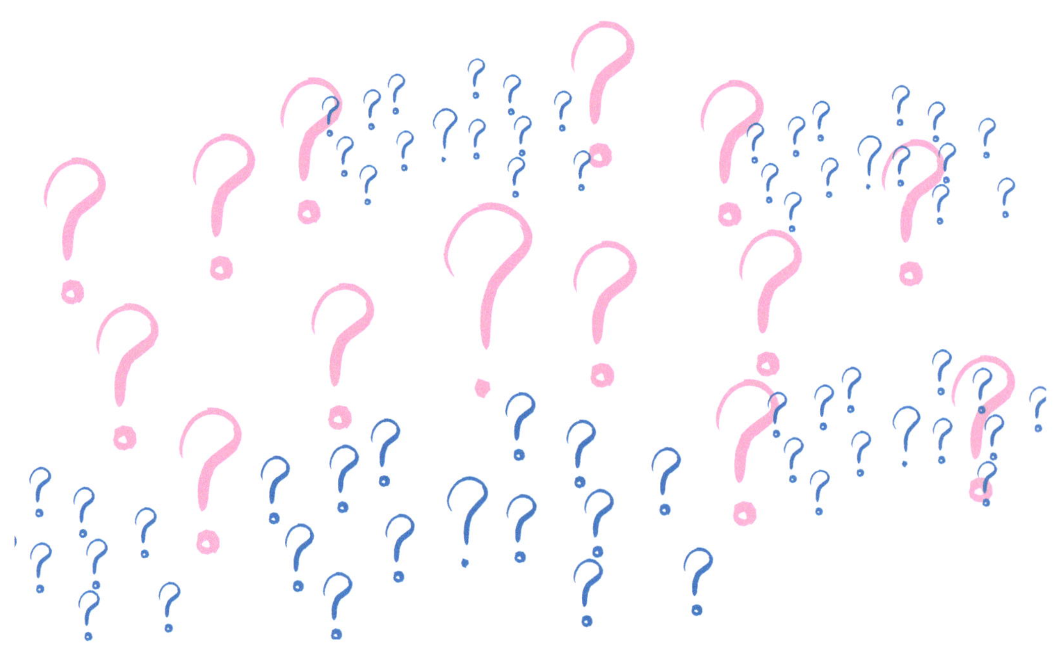

ASK YOURSELF, WHAT ONE THING COULD I DO
TODAY TO FEEL A LITTLE BETTER?

Day 4

BEGIN TODAY WITH GRATITUDE FOR YOUR BODY, AND WATCH IT RESPOND IN KIND.

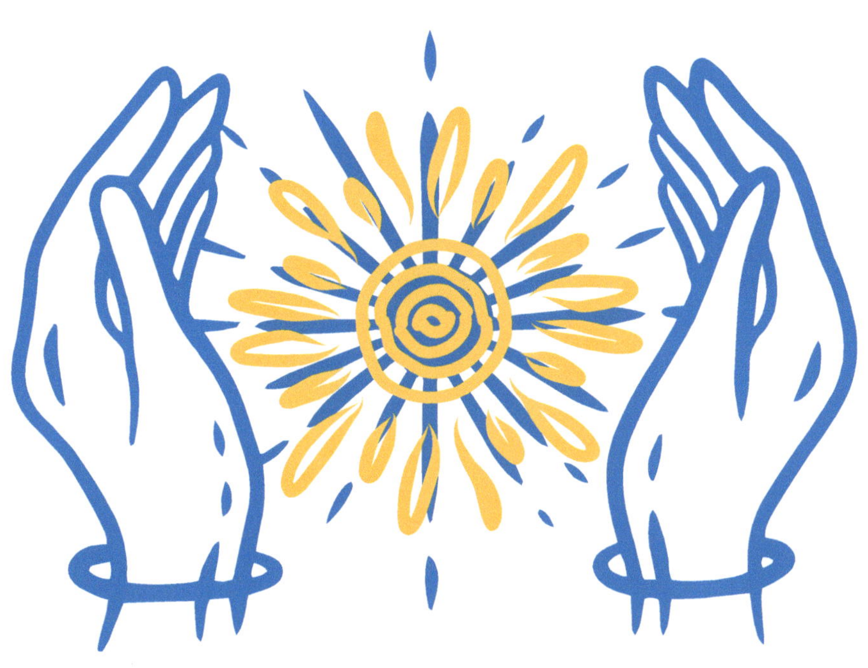

Day 5

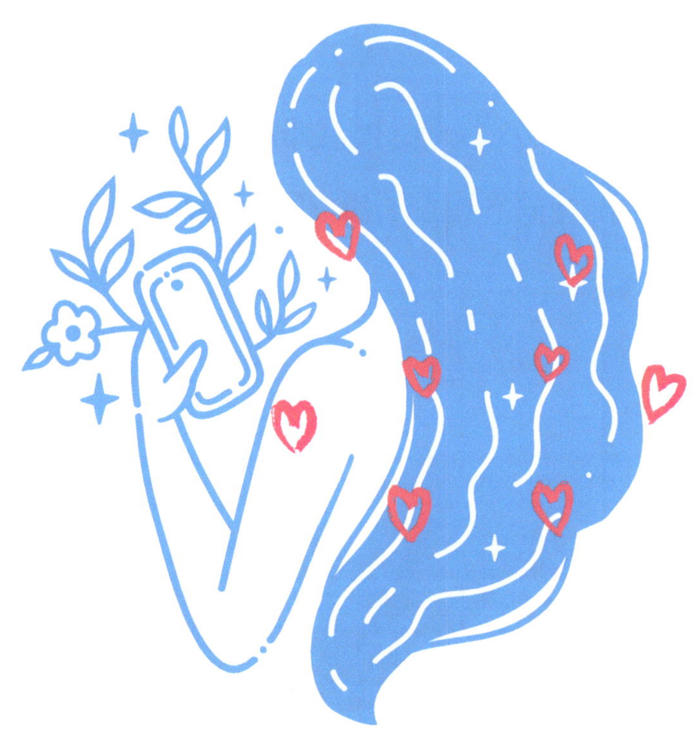

TRUE TRANSFORMATION BEGINS FROM THE INSIDE. START BY BEING KIND TO YOURSELF.

Day 6

START WITH ONE POSITIVE THOUGHT, AND LET IT GUIDE YOU THROUGH YOUR DAY.

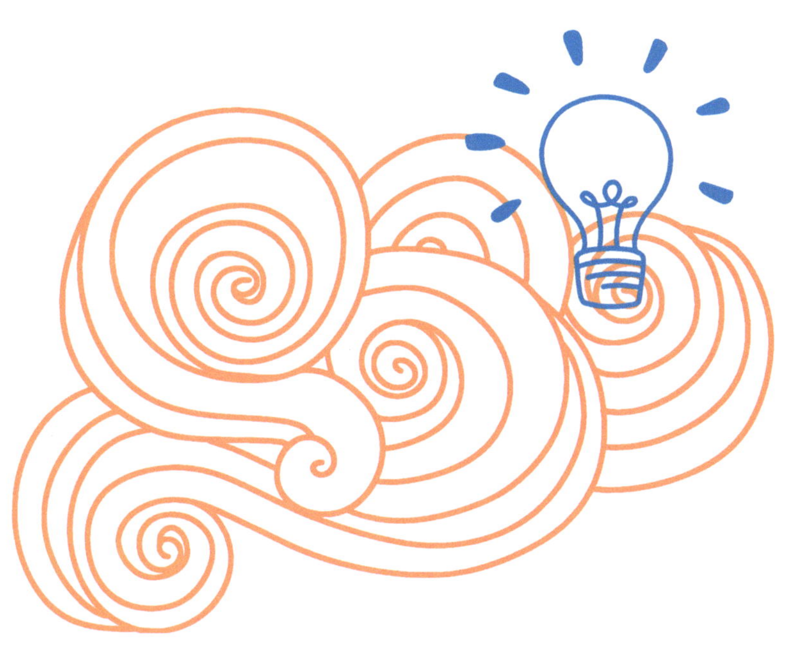

Day 7

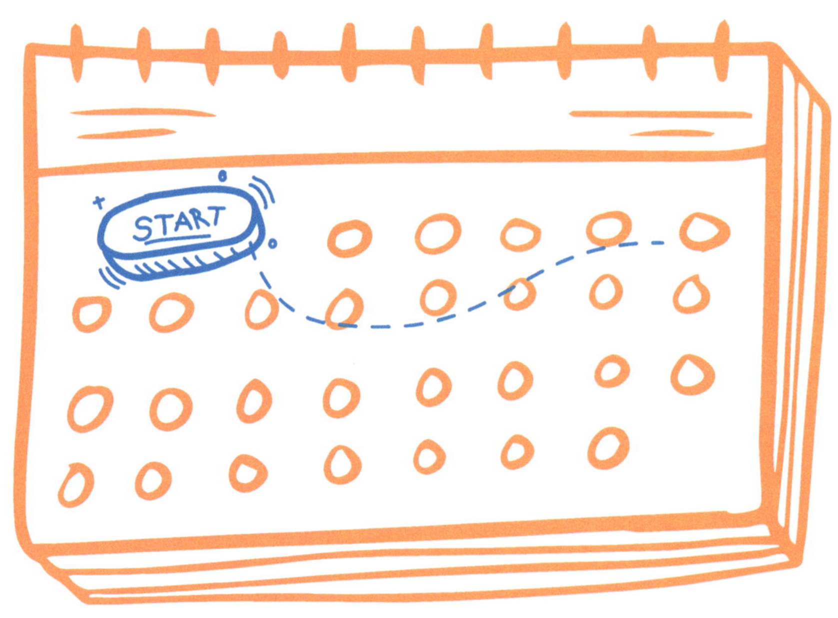

TO START, ALL YOU NEED IS THE DECISION TO
BE BETTER THAN YESTERDAY.

Day 8

THE MOST IMPORTANT THING YOU CAN DO FOR YOUR HEALTH TODAY IS TO BELIEVE IN YOUR ABILITY TO CHANGE.

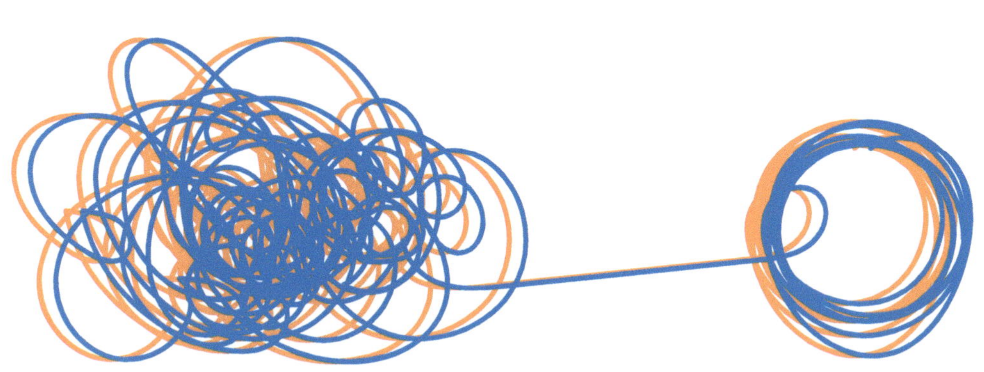

Day 9

IN THE QUIET MOMENTS, WE FIND CLARITY.
START TODAY WITH PEACE AND PURPOSE.

Day 10

HEALTH BEGINS IN YOUR MIND. WHEN YOU BELIEVE YOU DESERVE IT, YOU'LL MAKE IT HAPPEN.

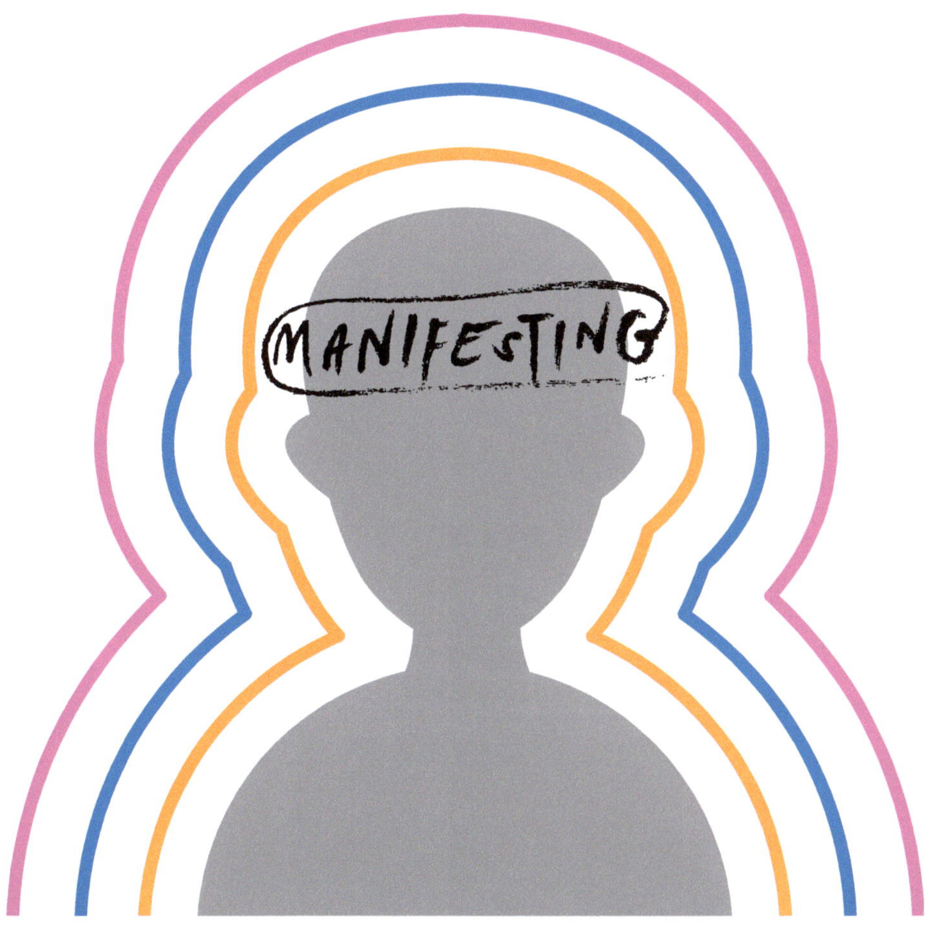

Notes

Eating for Health & Happiness

Nourish
with Love

2

Day 11

THINK OF YOUR MEALS AS A WAY TO FUEL YOUR DREAMS. WHEN YOU FEED YOUR BODY WELL, YOU FEED YOUR FUTURE.

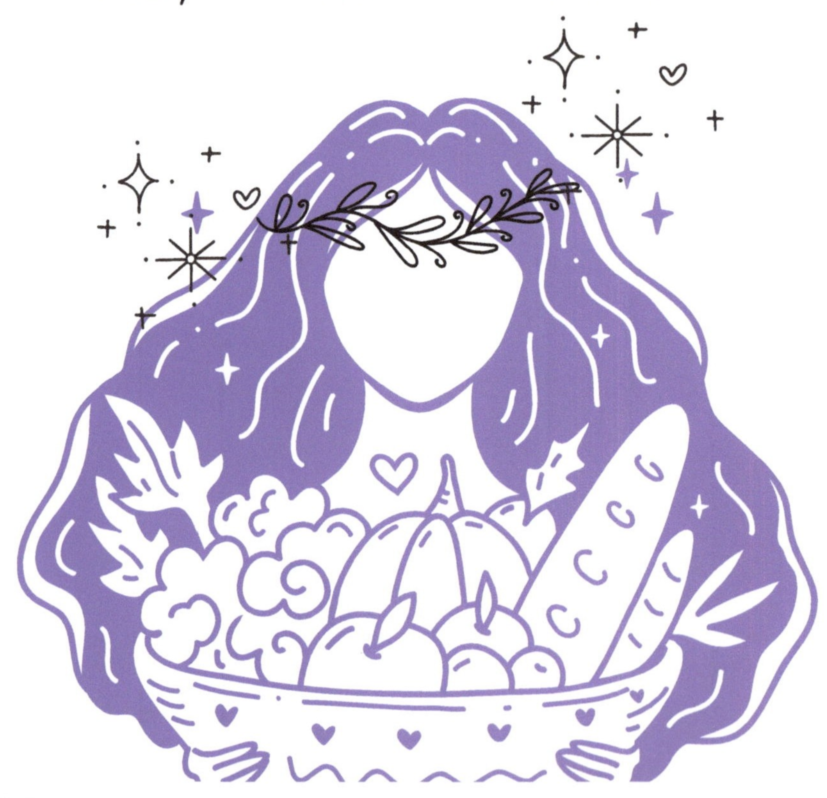

Day 12

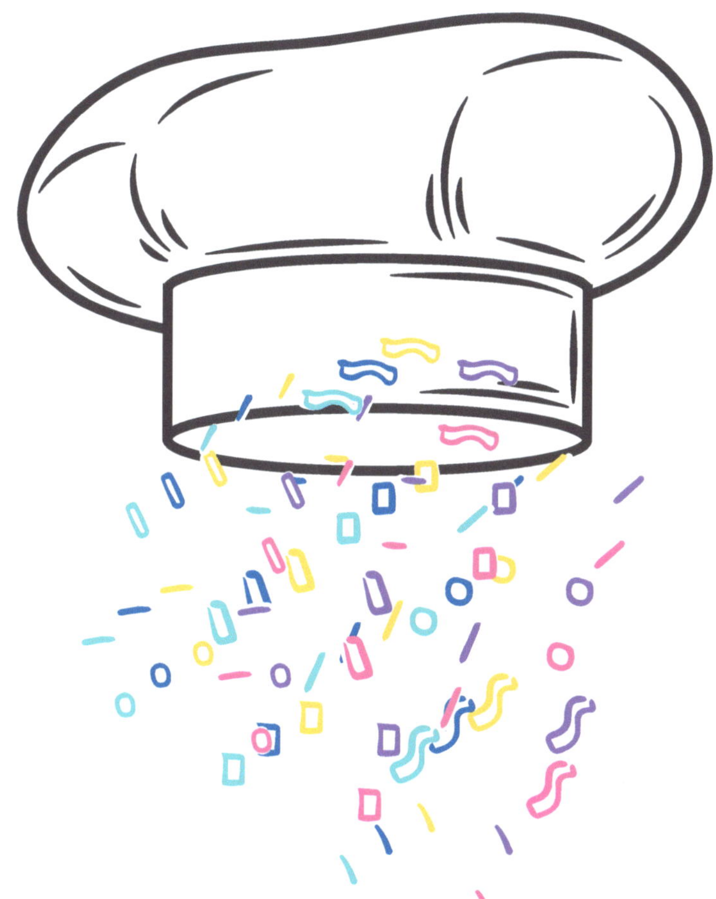

CELEBRATE FOOD THAT MAKES YOU FEEL VIBRANT. HEALTH STARTS WITH WHAT'S ON YOUR PLATE, BUT IT GROWS IN YOUR MIND.

Day 13

EATING WELL IS A FORM OF SELF-RESPECT. NOURISH YOUR BODY WITH LOVE, AND IT WILL RETURN THE FAVOR.

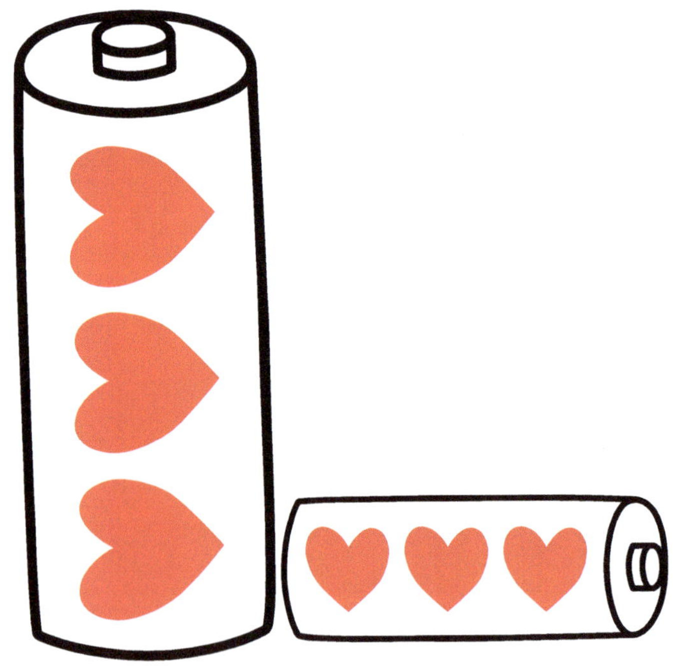

Day 14

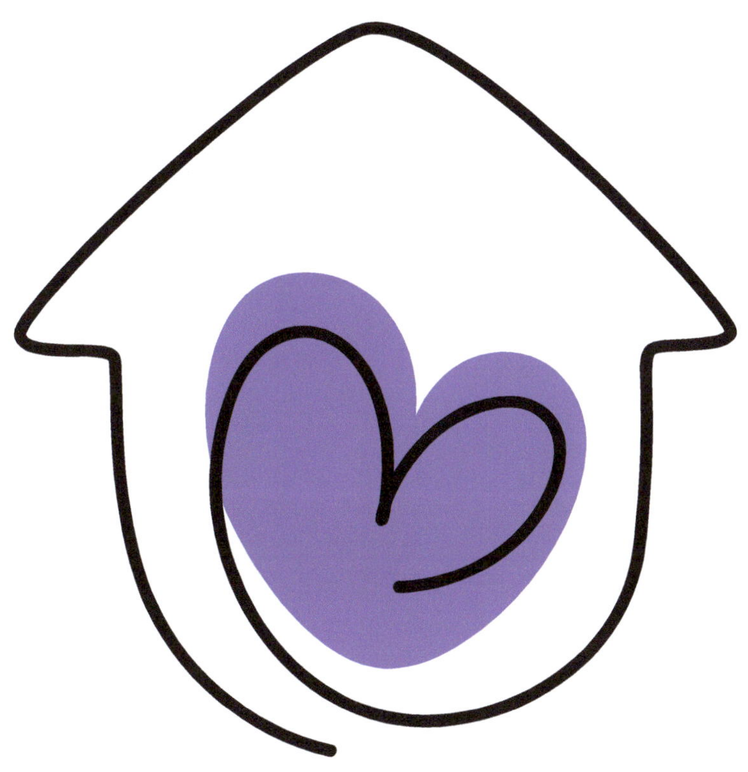

YOUR BODY IS YOUR HOME. FILL IT WITH THE NOURISHMENT IT DESERVES AND WATCH IT THRIVE.

Day 15

HEALTH ISN'T JUST ABOUT FOOD; IT'S ABOUT THE WAY YOU CARE FOR YOUR BODY, HEART, AND MIND.

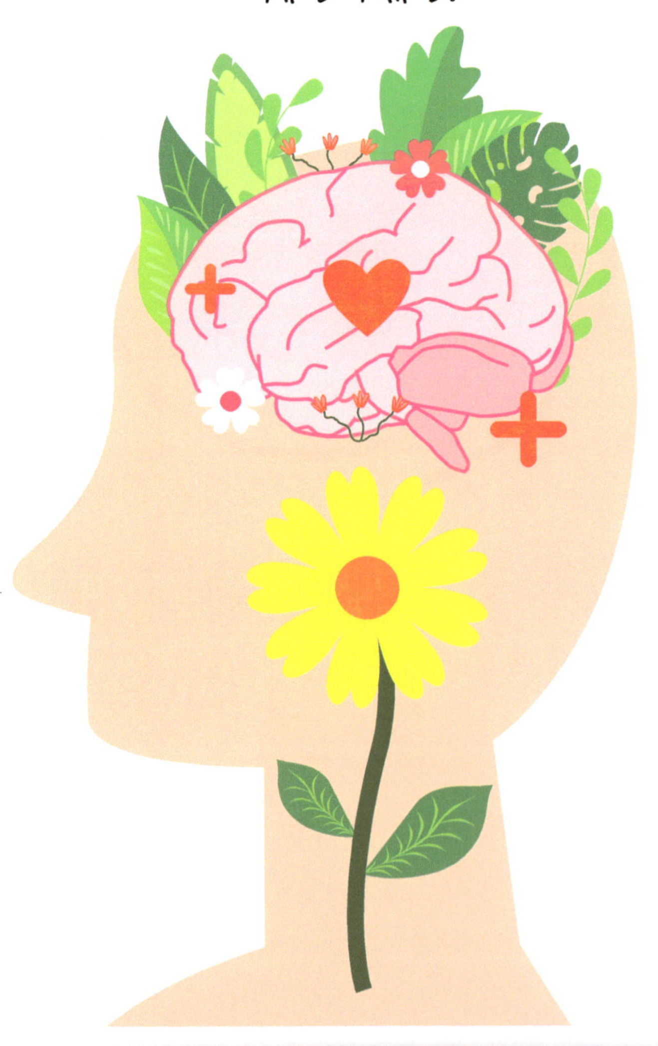

Day 16

EATING WITH LOVE MEANS CHOOSING FOODS THAT MAKE YOU FEEL ALIVE, ENERGIZED, AND AT PEACE..

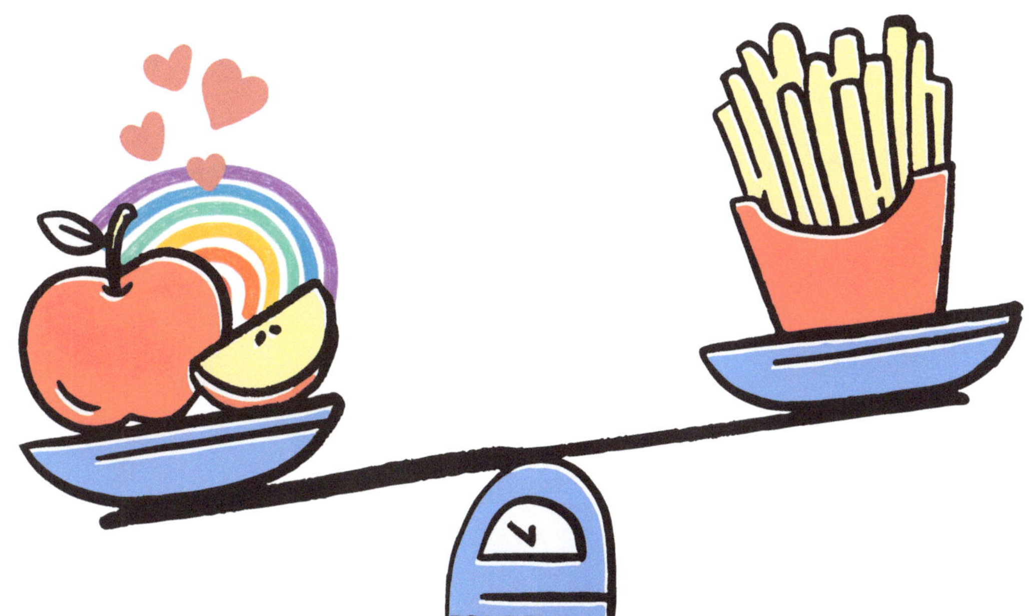

Day 17

LET FOOD BE THE MEDICINE THAT FUELS YOUR DREAMS, NOT THE BURDEN THAT WEIGHS YOU DOWN.

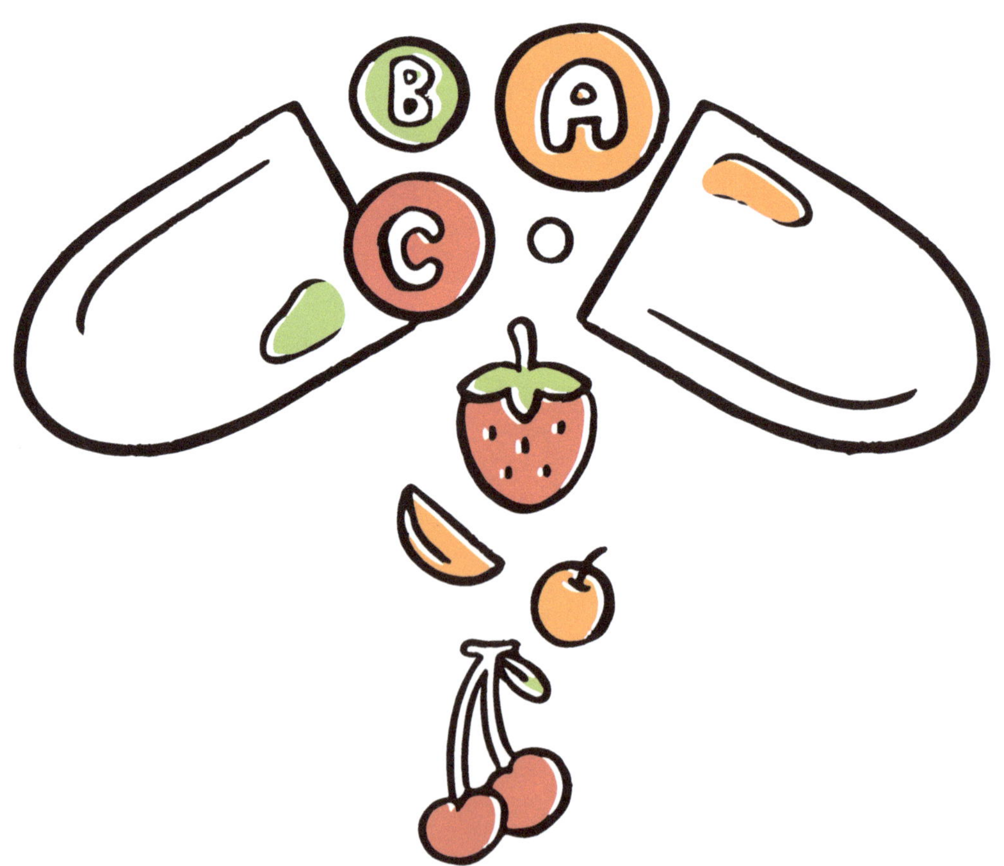

Day 18

NOURISH YOURSELF WITH WHOLESOME FOODS, AND WATCH THE JOY WITHIN YOU GROW.

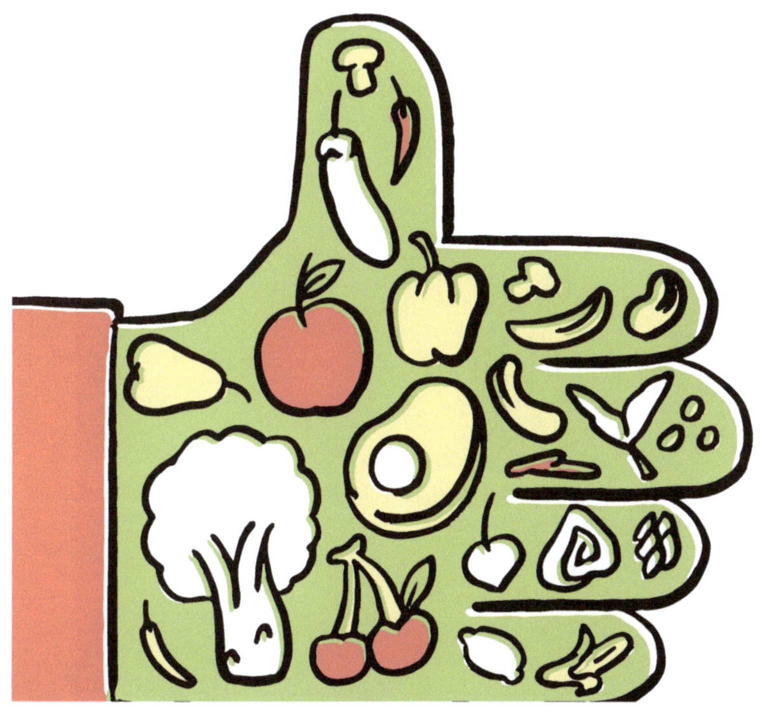

Day 19

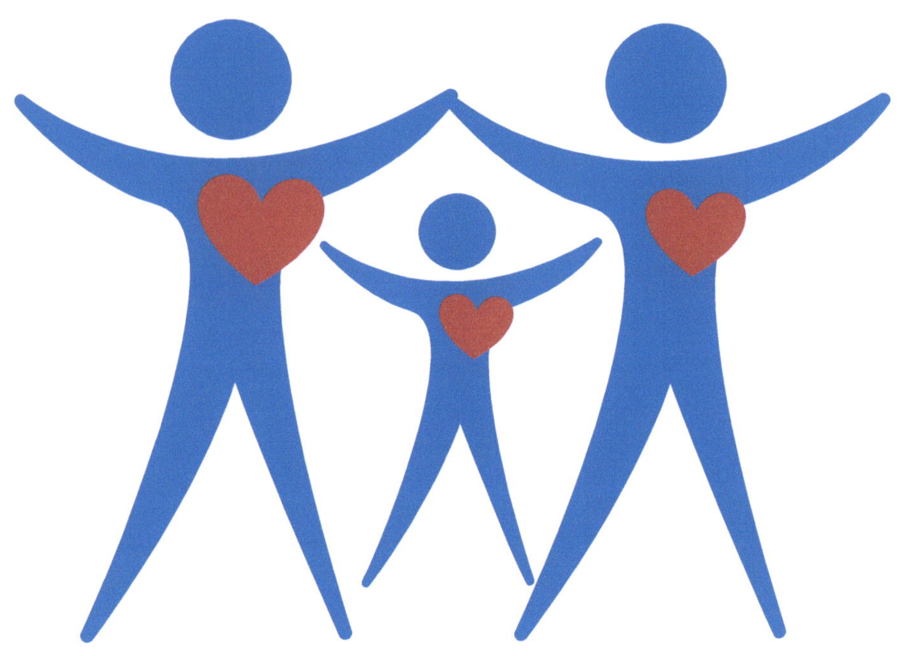

EVERY MEAL IS A CHANCE TO INVEST IN YOURSELF. CHOOSE LOVE, CHOOSE NOURISHMENT.

Day 20

FOOD IS NOT THE ENEMY; IT'S THE FUEL. FILL YOUR BODY WITH LOVE, AND YOU'LL FEEL UNSTOPPABLE.

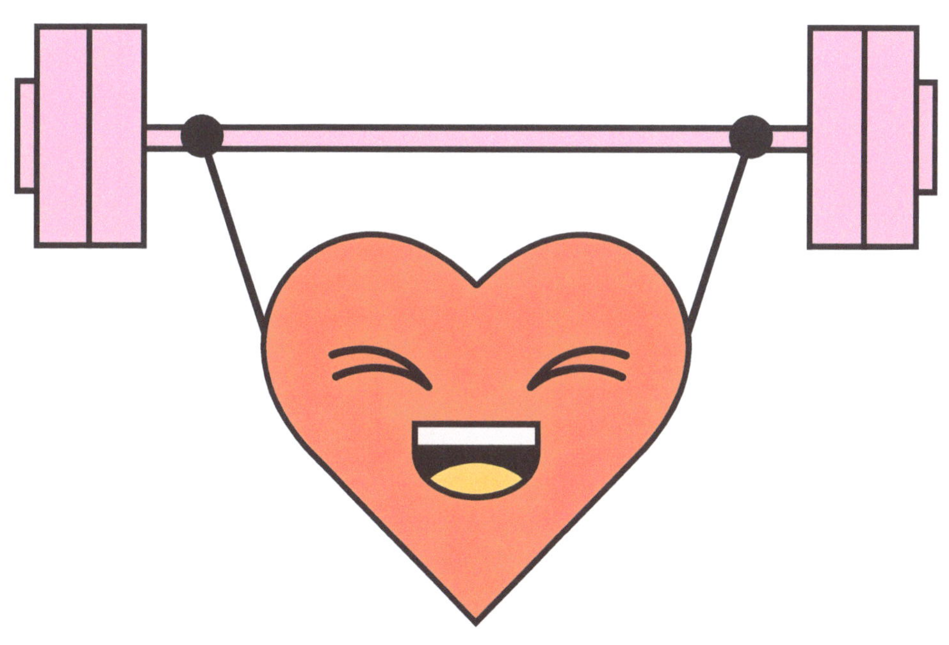

Day 21

WHEN YOU NOURISH YOUR BODY WITH LOVE,
YOU'RE NOT JUST FEEDING YOUR STOMACH,
YOU'RE FEEDING YOUR SOUL

Day 22

NOURISHING YOUR BODY IS THE ULTIMATE ACT OF GRATITUDE, FOR THE STRENGTH IT GIVES YOU TODAY AND THE POTENTIAL IT HOLDS FOR TOMORROW.

Notes

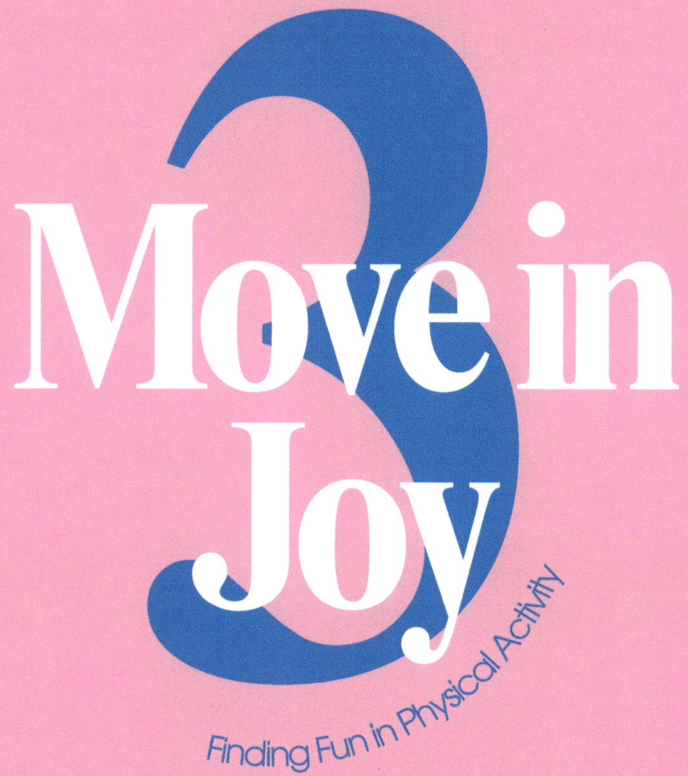

3
Move in Joy
Finding Fun in Physical Activity

Day 23

MOVEMENT ISN'T ABOUT BURNING CALORIES.
IT'S ABOUT CELEBRATING THE AMAZING
THINGS YOUR BODY CAN DO.

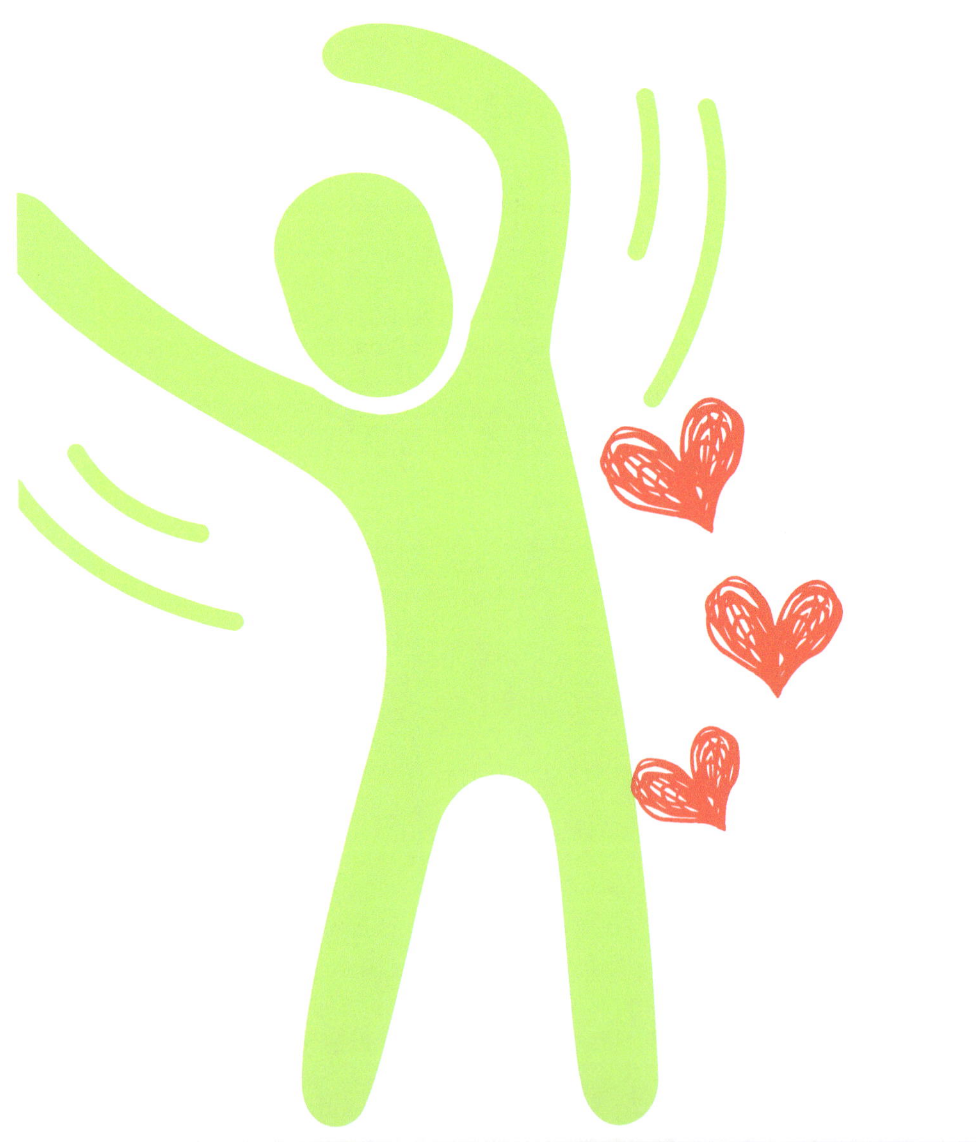

Day 24

MOVEMENT ISN'T ABOUT BURNING CALORIES. IT'S ABOUT CELEBRATING THE AMAZING THINGS YOUR BODY CAN DO.

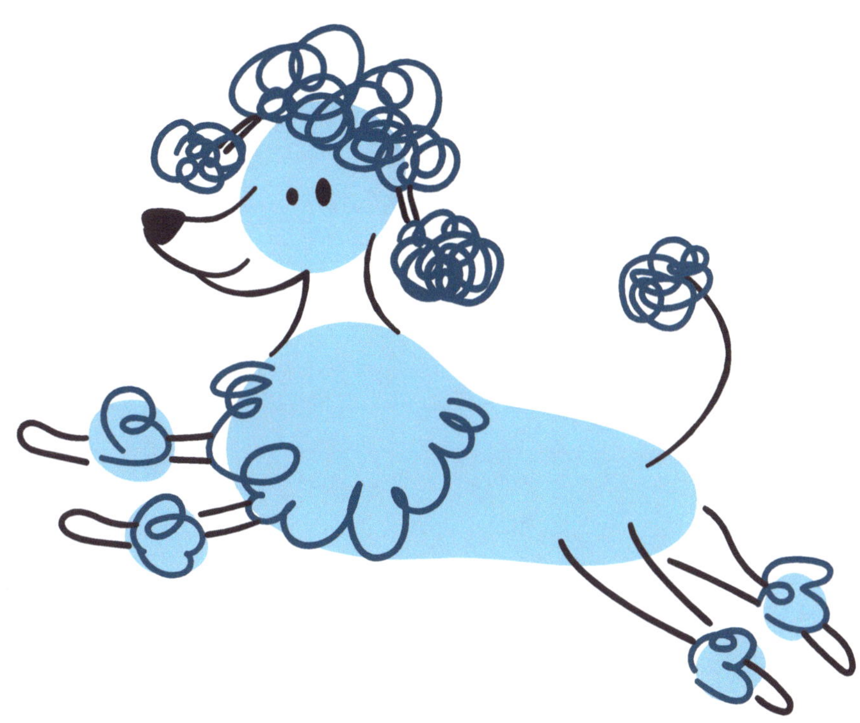

Day 25

THE BEST EXERCISE IS THE ONE THAT FEELS LIKE FREEDOM, NOT PUNISHMENT.

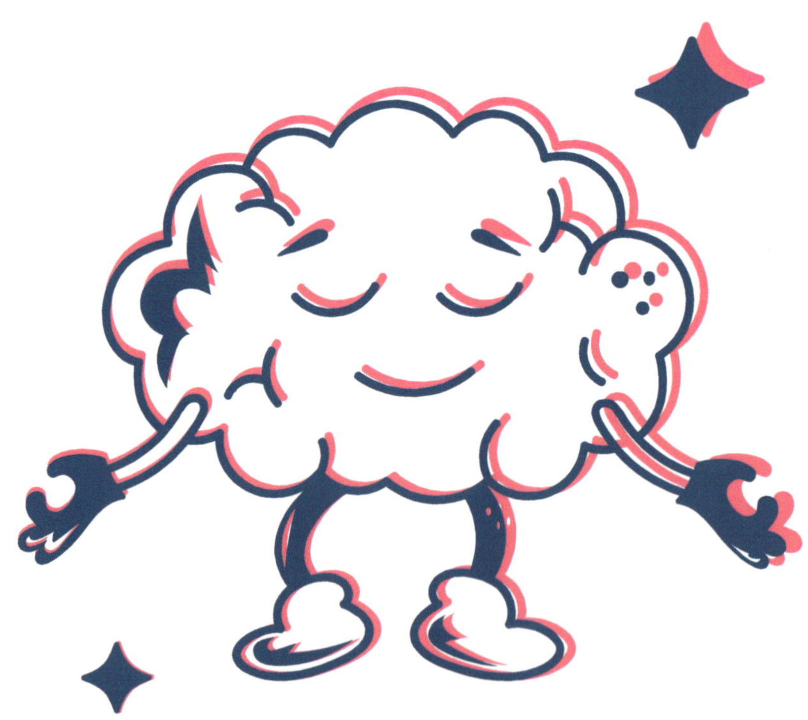

Day 26

STEP OUTSIDE, STRETCH, AND BREATHE.
SOMETIMES THE SIMPLEST MOVEMENTS BRING
THE GREATEST JOY.

Day 27

MOVE BECAUSE YOU LOVE YOUR BODY, NOT BECAUSE YOU'RE TRYING TO CHANGE IT.

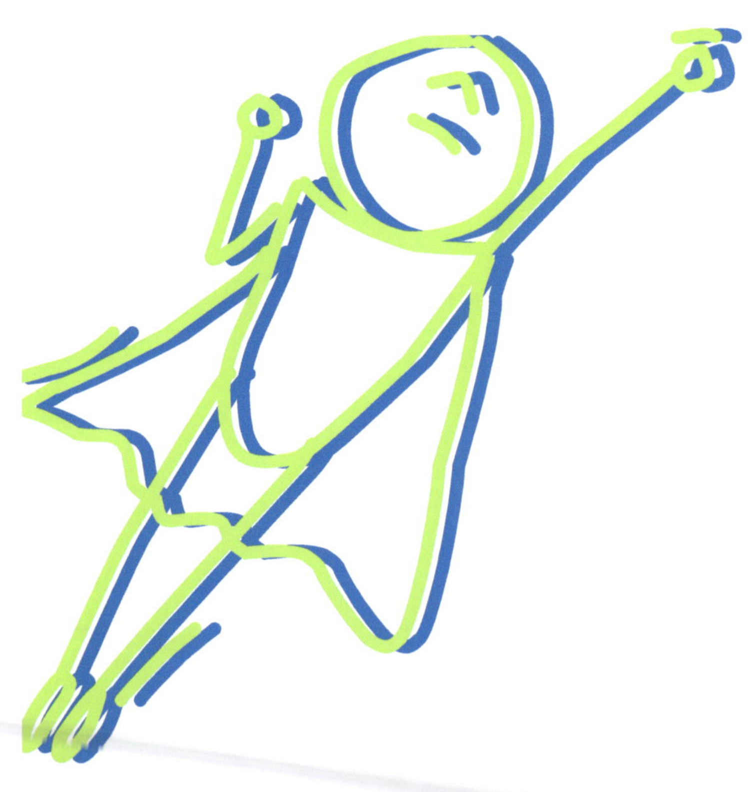

Day 28

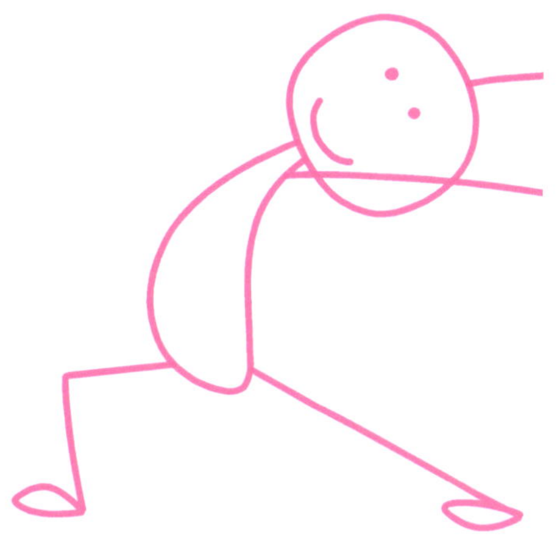

THINK OF MOVEMENT AS PLAY, NOT WORK.
DANCE, STRETCH, EXPLORE. LET IT BE FUN!

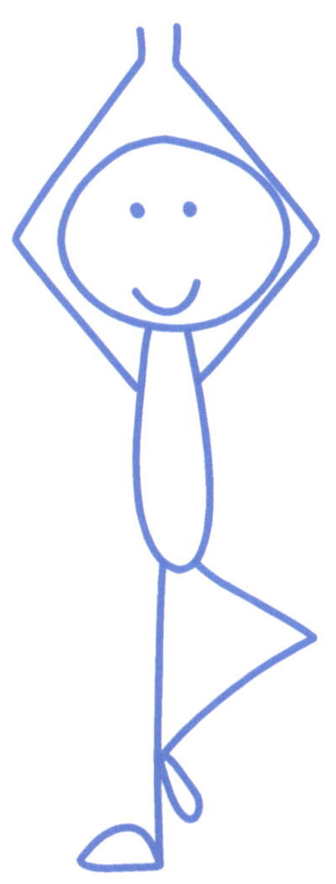

Day 29

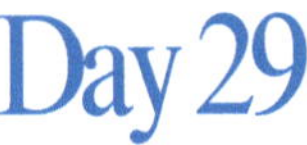

EVERY STEP, EVERY STRETCH, EVERY JUMP IS
A CELEBRATION OF LIFE AND ENERGY.

Day 30

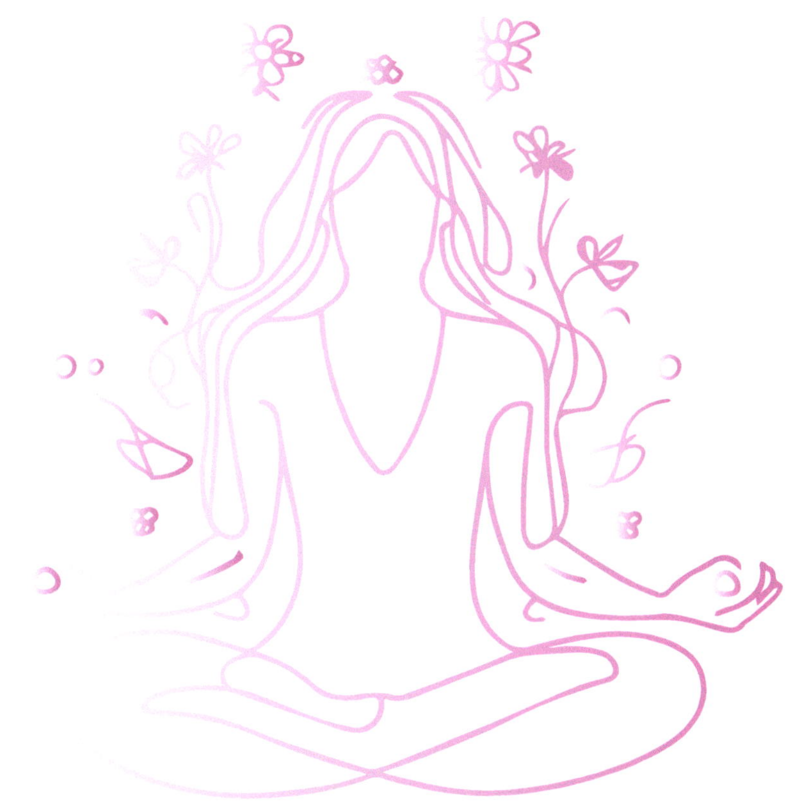

YOUR BODY IS A MIRACLE, TREAT IT TO THE
JOY OF MOVING FREELY.

Day 31

EXERCISE ISN'T A TASK; IT'S A GIFT YOU GIVE TO YOURSELF. A REMINDER OF YOUR STRENGTH AND VITALITY.

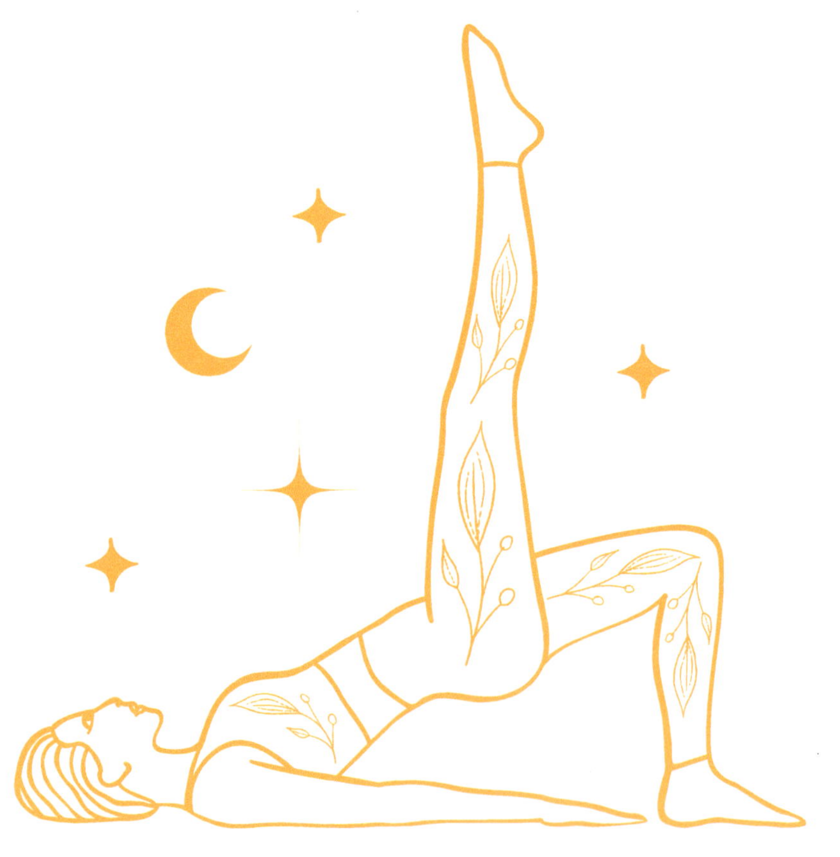

Day 32

FIND THE RHYTHM THAT FEELS LIKE YOU. MOVEMENT ISN'T ONE-SIZE-FITS-ALL. IT'S AN EXPRESSION OF YOUR JOY.

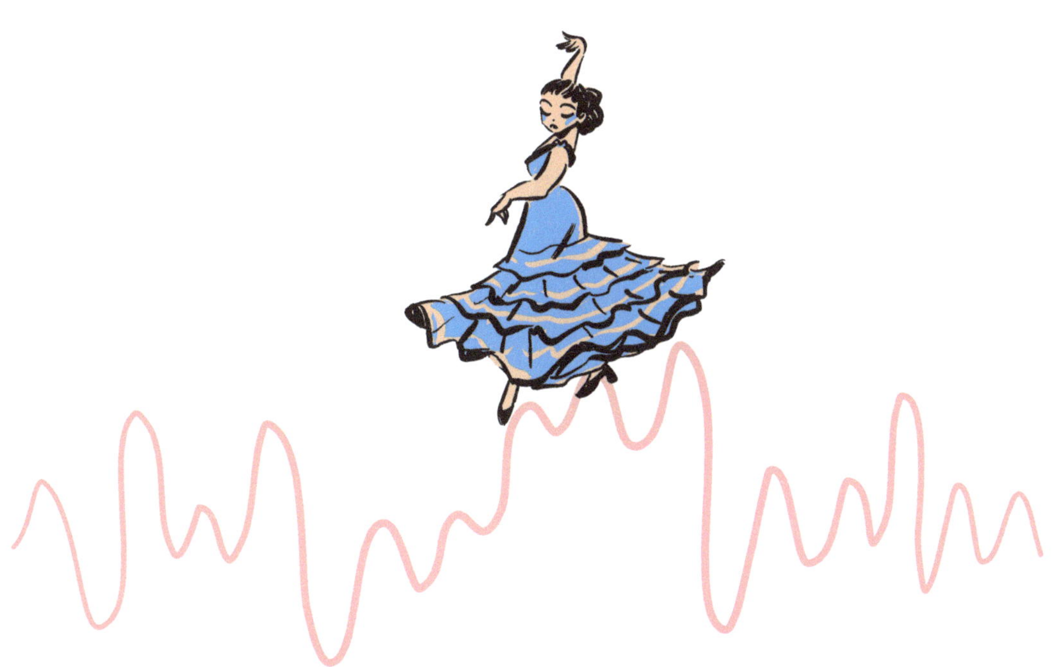

Day 33

YOU DON'T NEED A GYM TO MOVE YOUR BODY. ALL YOU NEED IS A LITTLE CURIOSITY AND THE WILL TO BEGIN.

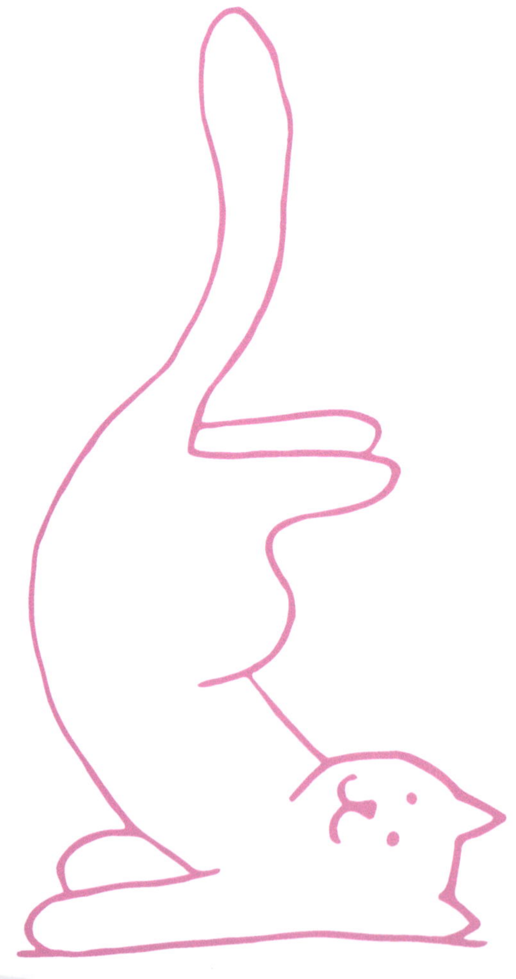

Notes

Notes

The Power of Pause

Day 34

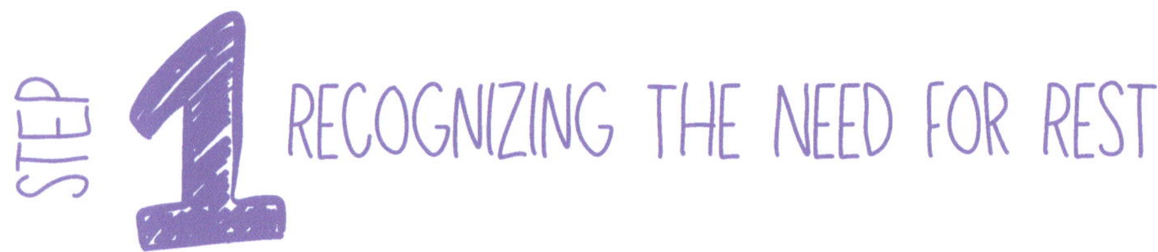

EXHAUSTION ISN'T A BADGE OF HONOR. IT'S YOUR BODY'S WAY OF ASKING FOR CARE.

Understand that needing rest is natural and essential.

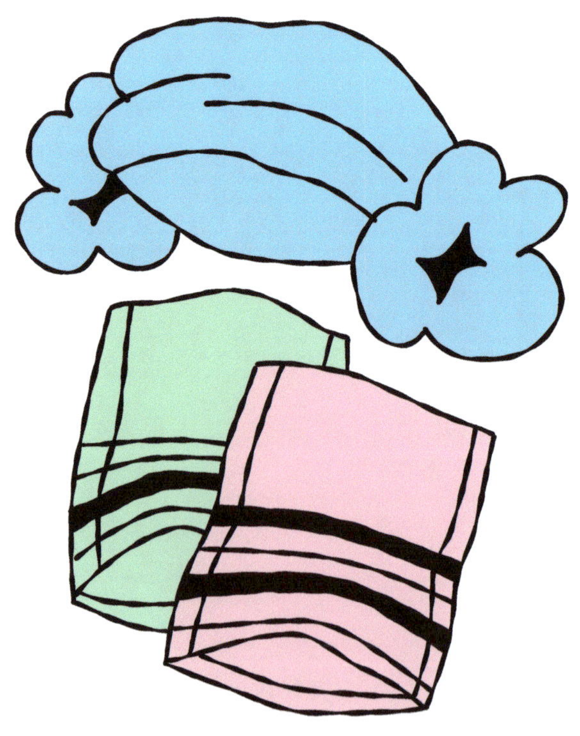

Day 35

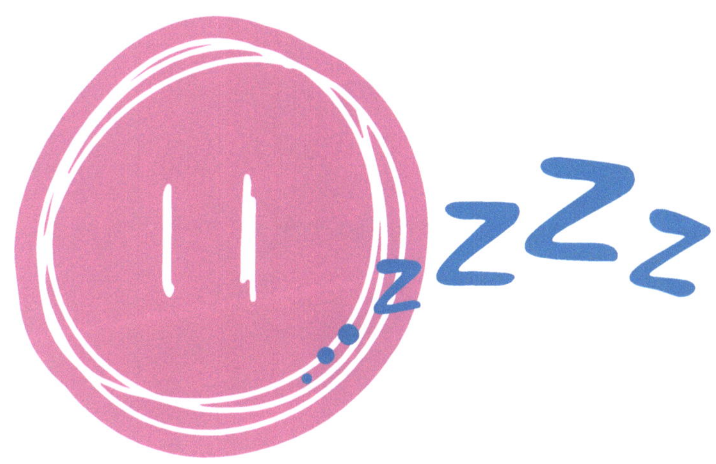

PAUSE. YOUR WORTH ISN'T TIED TO HOW MUCH YOU DO BUT TO HOW WELL YOU CARE FOR YOURSELF.

Shift your mindset about the importance of taking breaks

STEP 2 GIVING YOURSELF PERMISSION TO PAUSE

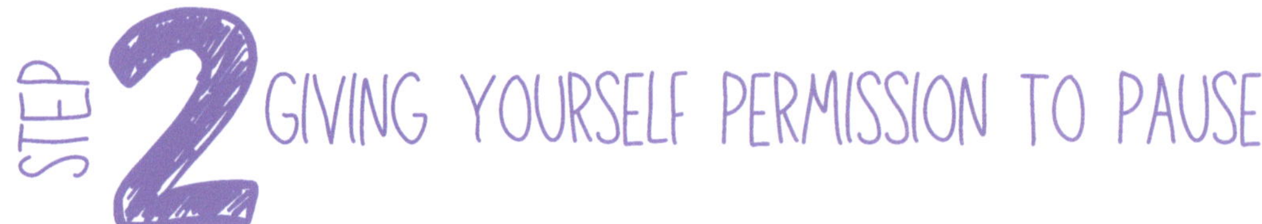

REST IS PRODUCTIVE. IT'S THE QUIET ENERGY THAT POWERS YOUR NEXT LEAP FORWARD.

Reframe rest as a crucial part of achievement.

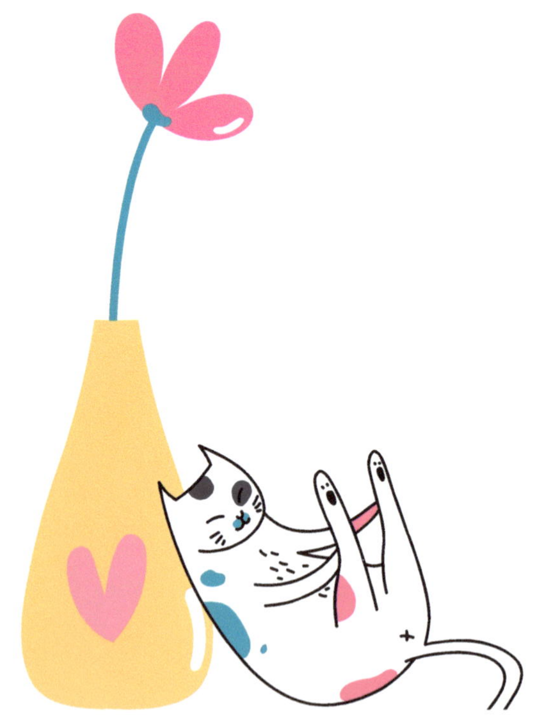

STEP **2** GIVING YOURSELF PERMISSION TO PAUSE

YOU DON'T NEED TO EARN REST. IT'S YOUR RIGHT AS A HUMAN BEING.

Let go of guilt and embrace rest as a necessity, not a reward.

Day 38

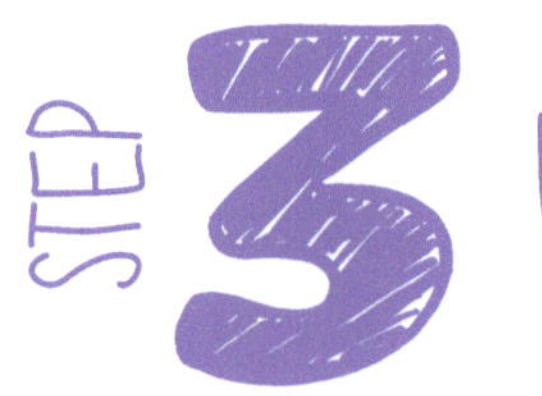

3 EMBRACING REST AS SELF-CARE

SLEEP IS YOUR SUPERPOWER. EVERY NIGHT, YOUR BODY RESETS, HEALS, AND PREPARES FOR GREATNESS.

Focus on the restorative magic of sleep.

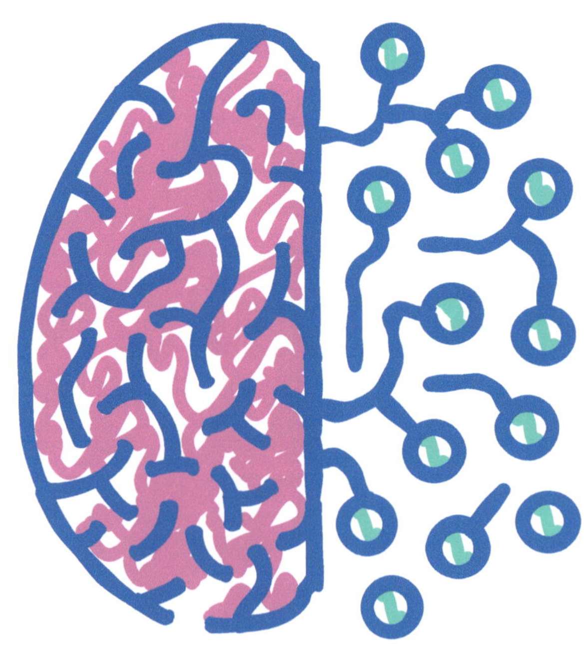

Day 39

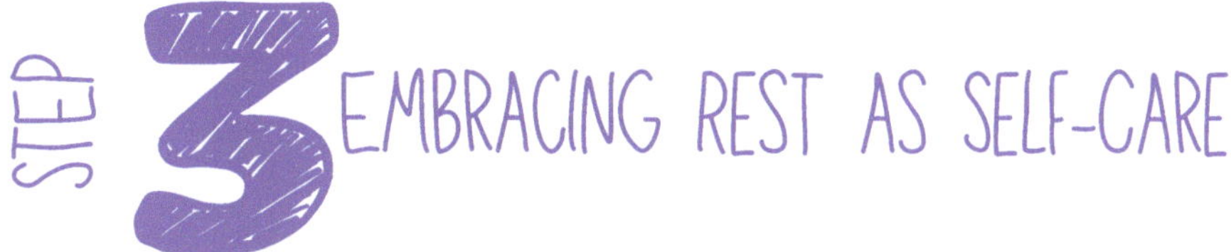

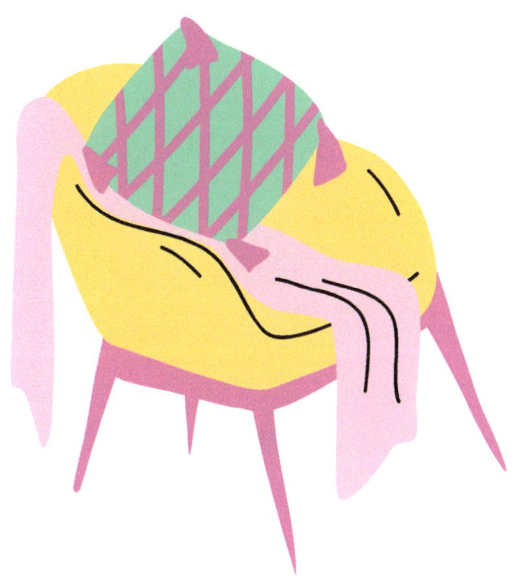

A RESTED BODY CREATES A CLEAR MIND. WHEN YOU PAUSE, YOU ALLOW CLARITY TO FLOW IN.

Highlight the mental benefits of recharging.

STEP 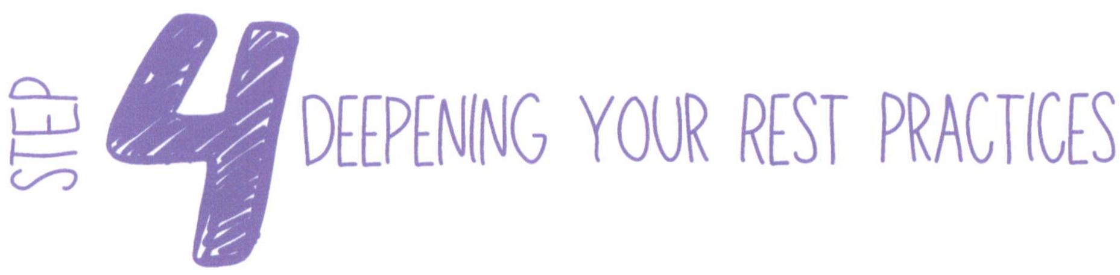 4 DEEPENING YOUR REST PRACTICES

TRUE REST IS MORE THAN SLEEP. IT'S THE ART OF LETTING YOUR MIND AND SOUL FIND PEACE.

Encourage exploring deeper ways to rest, like mindfulness or solitude.

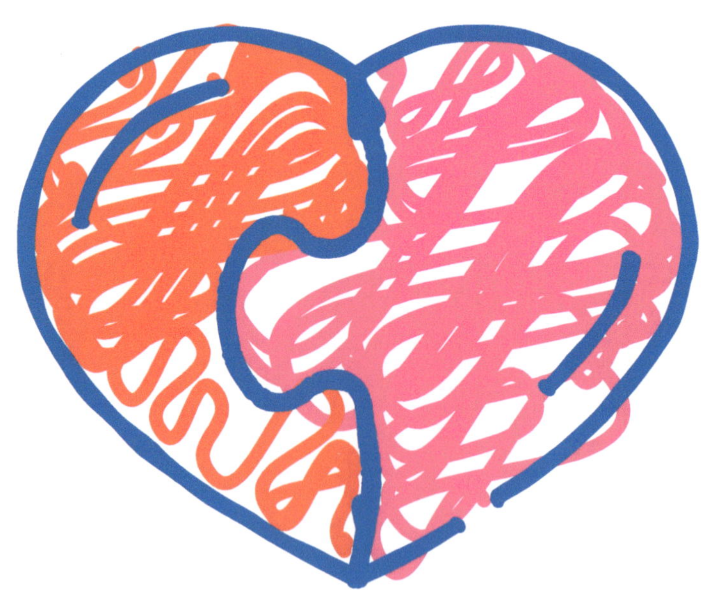

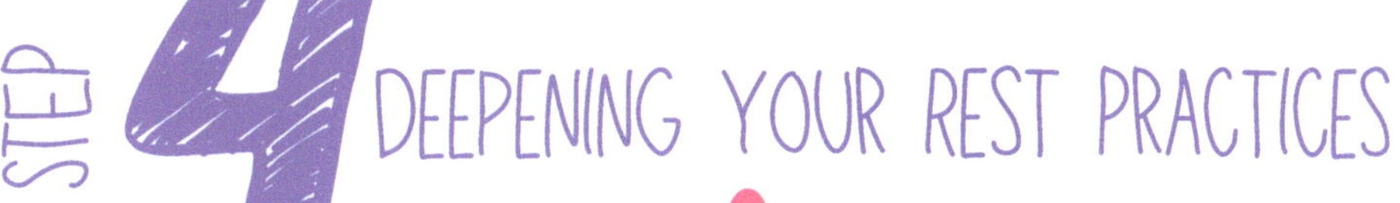

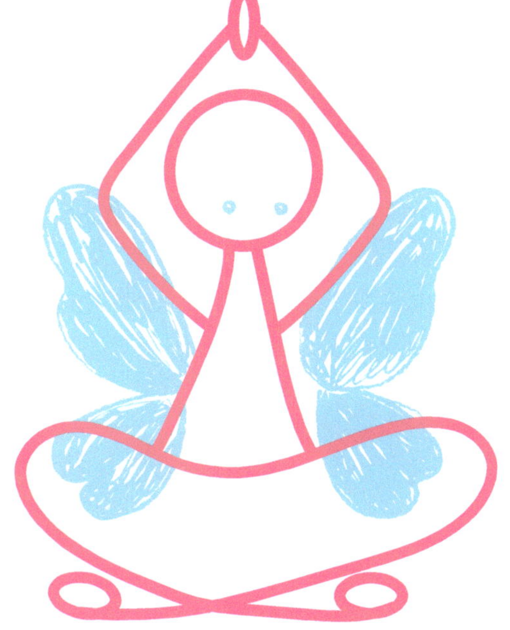

BREATHE IN CALM, EXHALE TENSION. EACH MOMENT OF STILLNESS IS A STEP TOWARD RENEWAL.

Introduce breathing as a quick, restorative pause.

Day 42

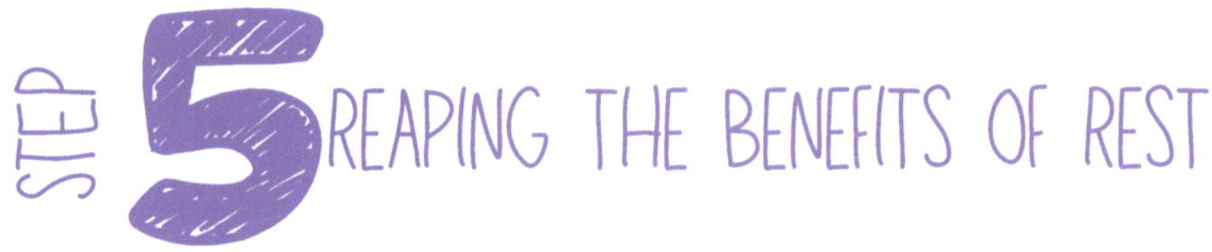

WHEN YOU HONOR REST, YOU GIFT YOURSELF THE ENERGY TO LIVE FULLY.

Celebrate the transformation rest brings to your energy and focus.

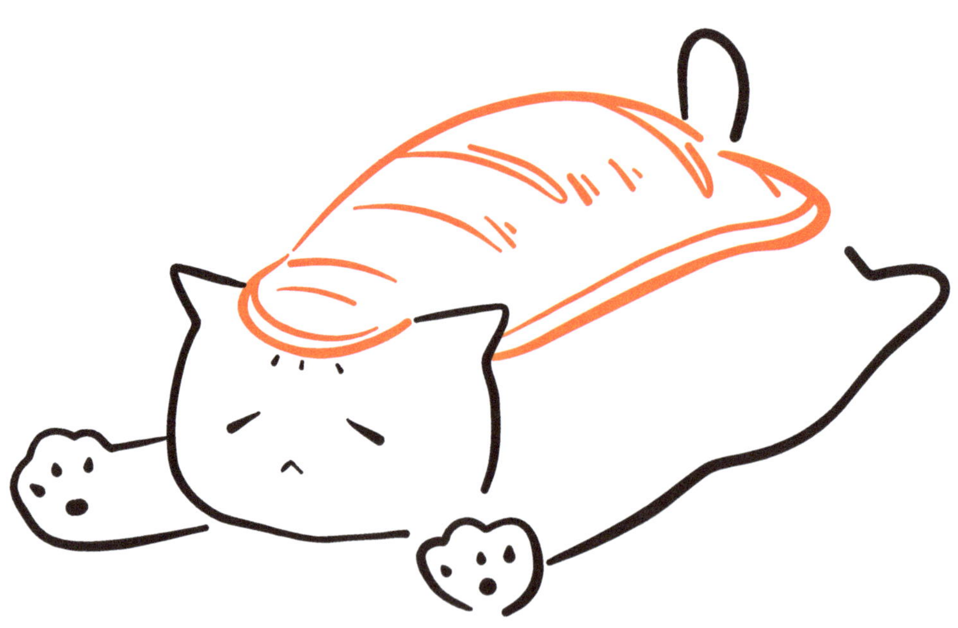

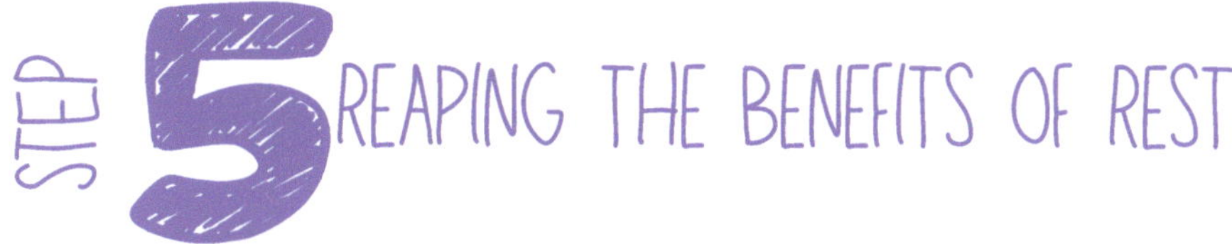

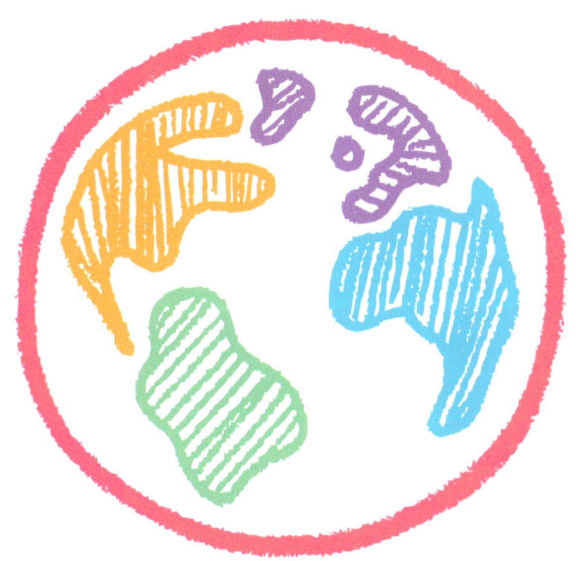

THE WORLD MOVES FAST, BUT YOU DON'T HAVE TO. REST ALLOWS YOU TO SAVOR LIFE, NOT JUST SURVIVE IT.

Inspire you to find joy in slowing down and recharging.

Notes

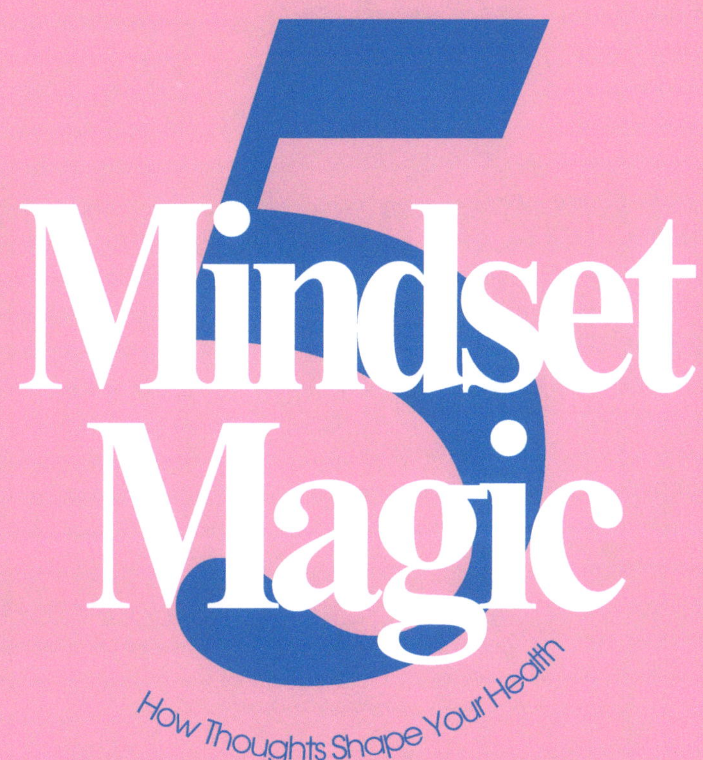

5
Mindset
Magic
How Thoughts Shape Your Health

Day 44

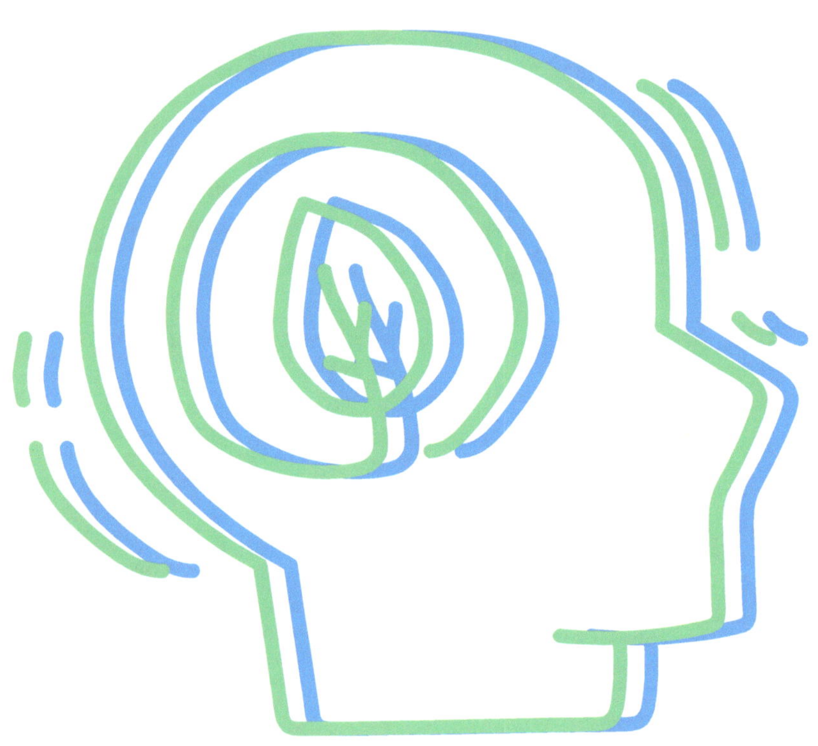

THE JOURNEY TO HEALTH BEGINS IN YOUR MIND. SHIFT YOUR FOCUS FROM WHAT'S WRONG TO EVERYTHING THAT'S POSSIBLE.

Day 45

YOUR THOUGHTS ARE THE SEEDS OF YOUR REALITY. PLANT HOPE, WATER IT WITH ACTION, AND WATCH YOUR HEALTH FLOURISH.

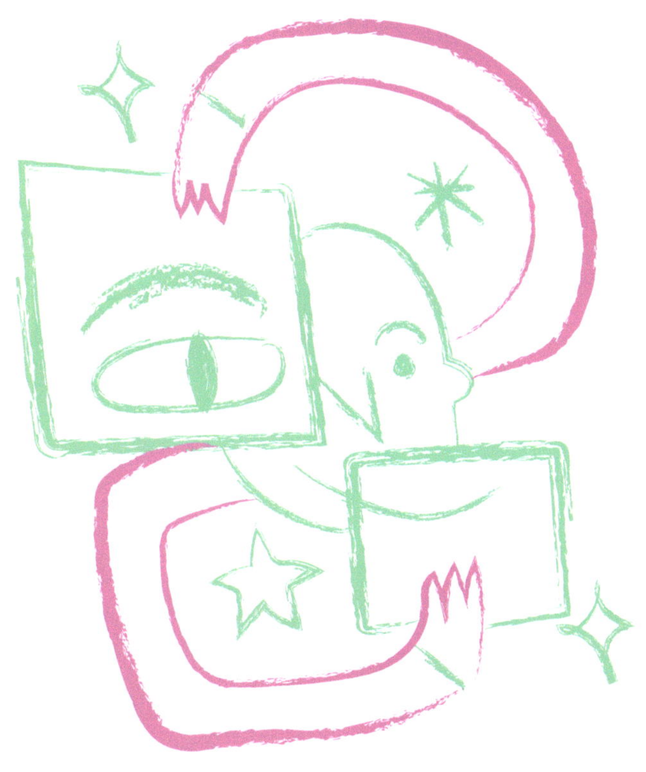

Day 46

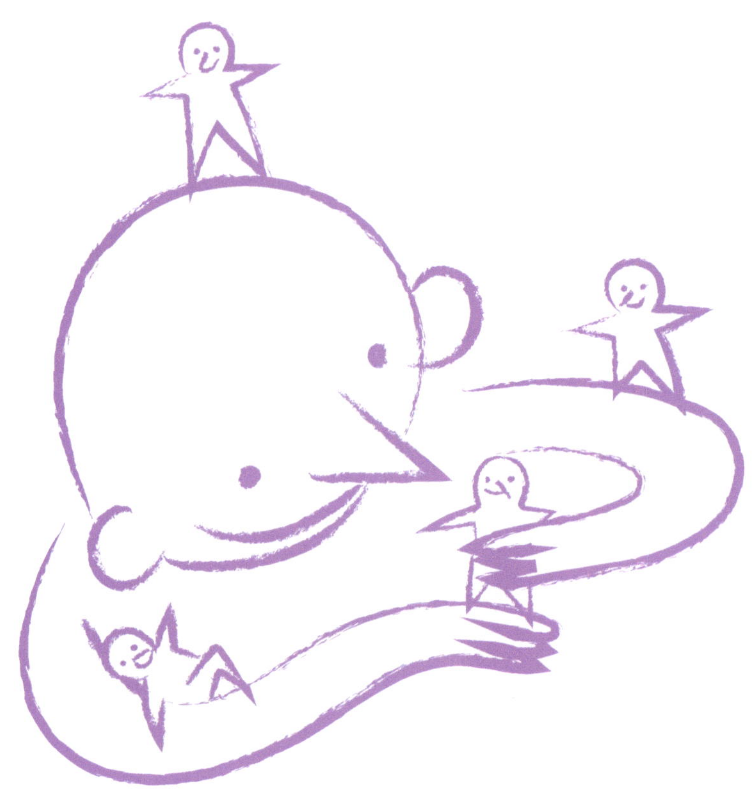

WHAT YOU TELL YOURSELF MATTERS. SPEAK WORDS OF ENCOURAGEMENT, NOT CRITICISM, AND SEE THE CHANGE IT INSPIRES.

Day 47

YOUR MINDSET SHAPES YOUR HABITS, AND YOUR HABITS BUILD YOUR LIFE. START WITH A BELIEF IN YOUR ABILITY TO THRIVE.

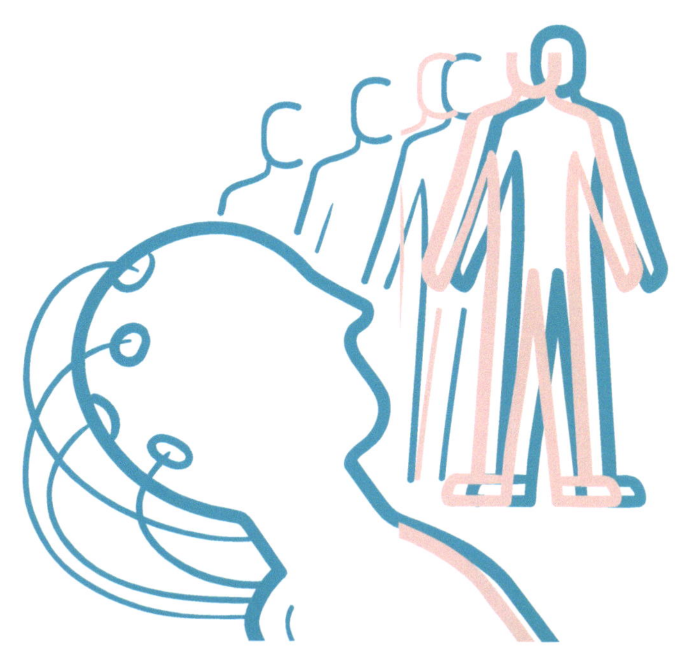

Day 48

SEE CHALLENGES AS OPPORTUNITIES. EACH OBSTACLE IS A CHANCE TO GROW STRONGER AND CLOSER TO YOUR HEALTHIEST SELF.

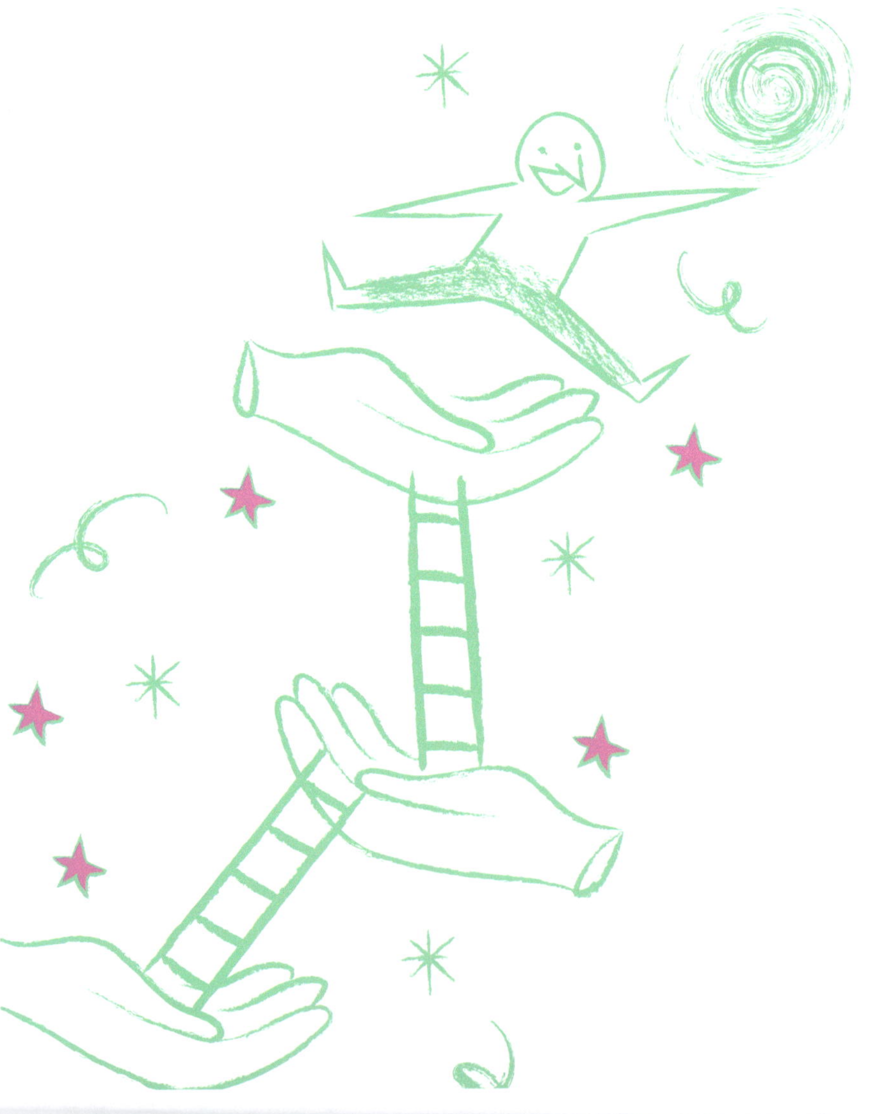

Day 49

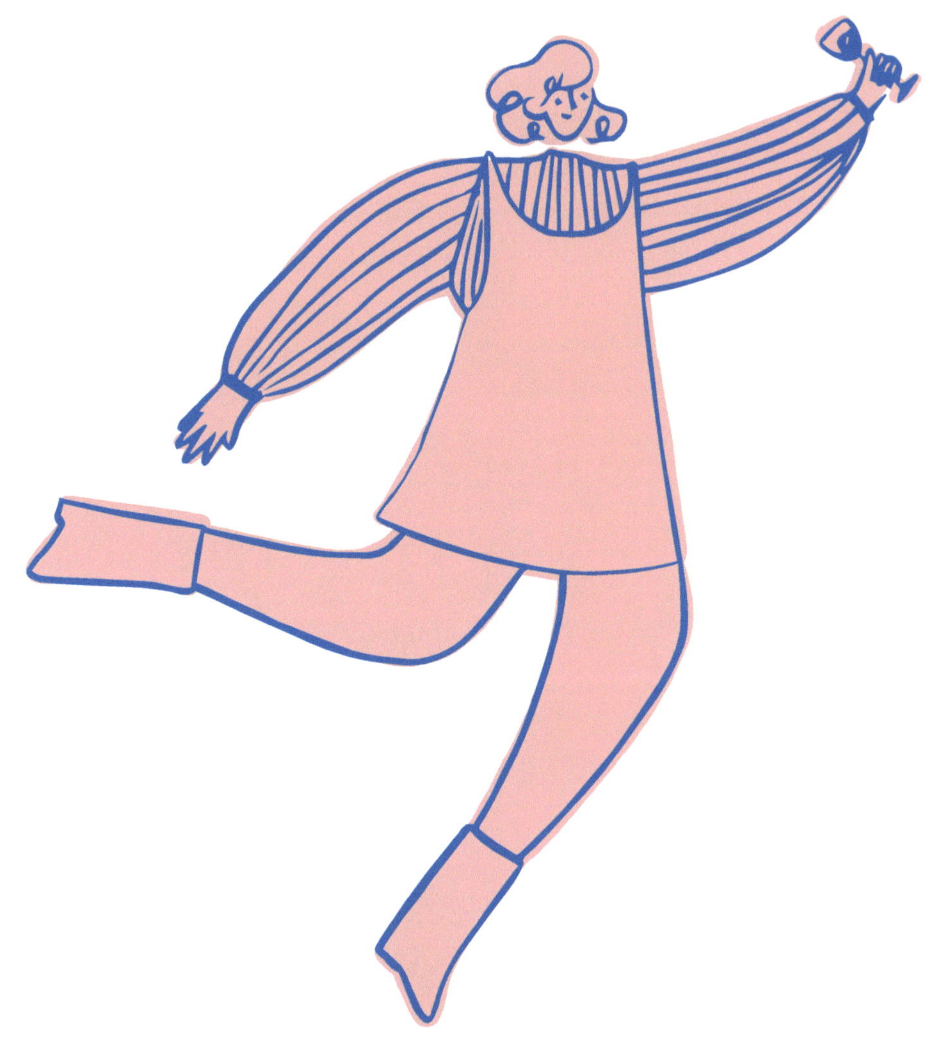

CELEBRATE PROGRESS, NOT PERFECTION. EVERY SMALL WIN IS A STEP TOWARD THE BIGGER PICTURE..

Day 50

RELEASE THE NEED TO COMPARE. YOUR HEALTH JOURNEY IS UNIQUELY YOURS. HONOR IT.

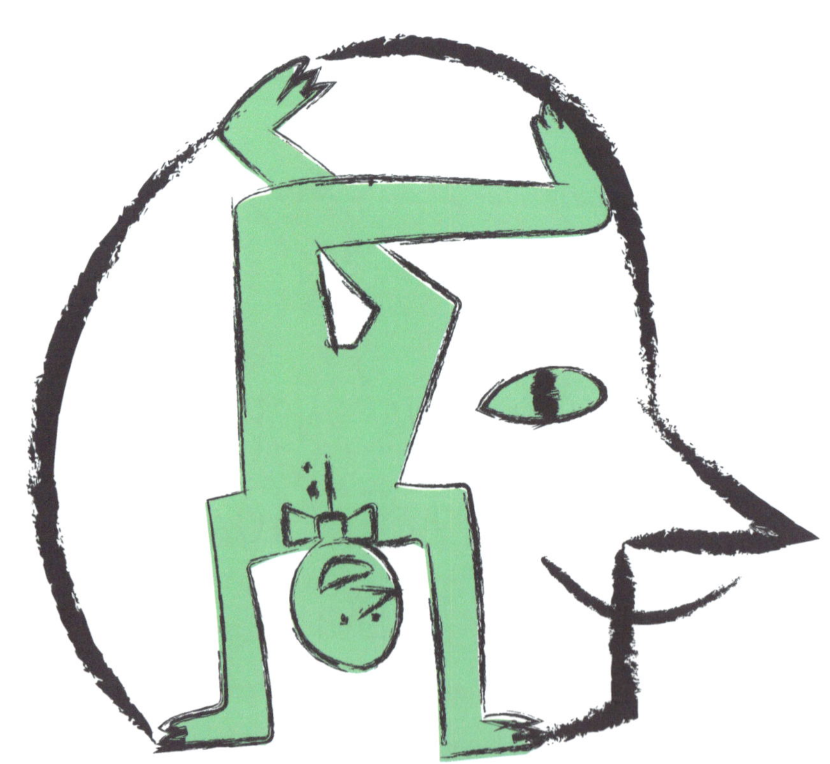

Day 51

VISUALIZE YOUR HEALTHIEST SELF. NOT JUST HOW YOU LOOK, BUT HOW YOU FEEL. USE THAT VISION AS YOUR GUIDE.

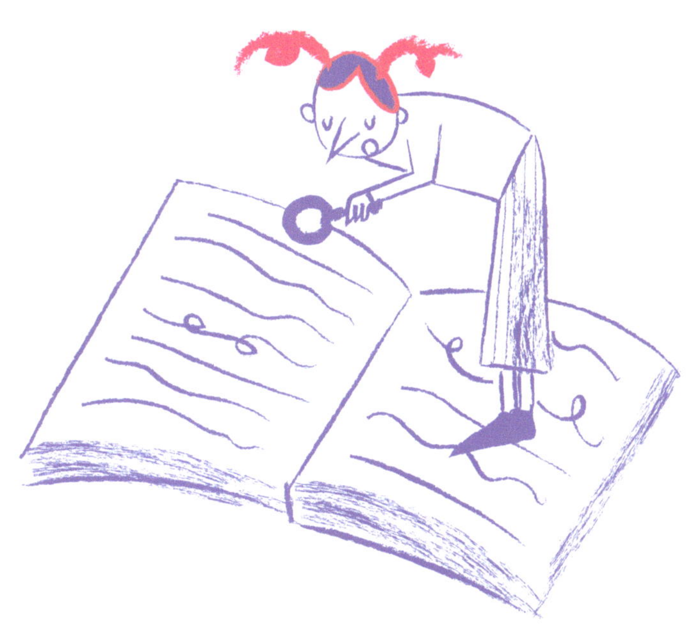

Day 52

TRUST THE PROCESS, EVEN WHEN IT FEELS SLOW. CONSISTENT POSITIVITY AND EFFORT CREATE THE RESULTS YOU DESIRE.

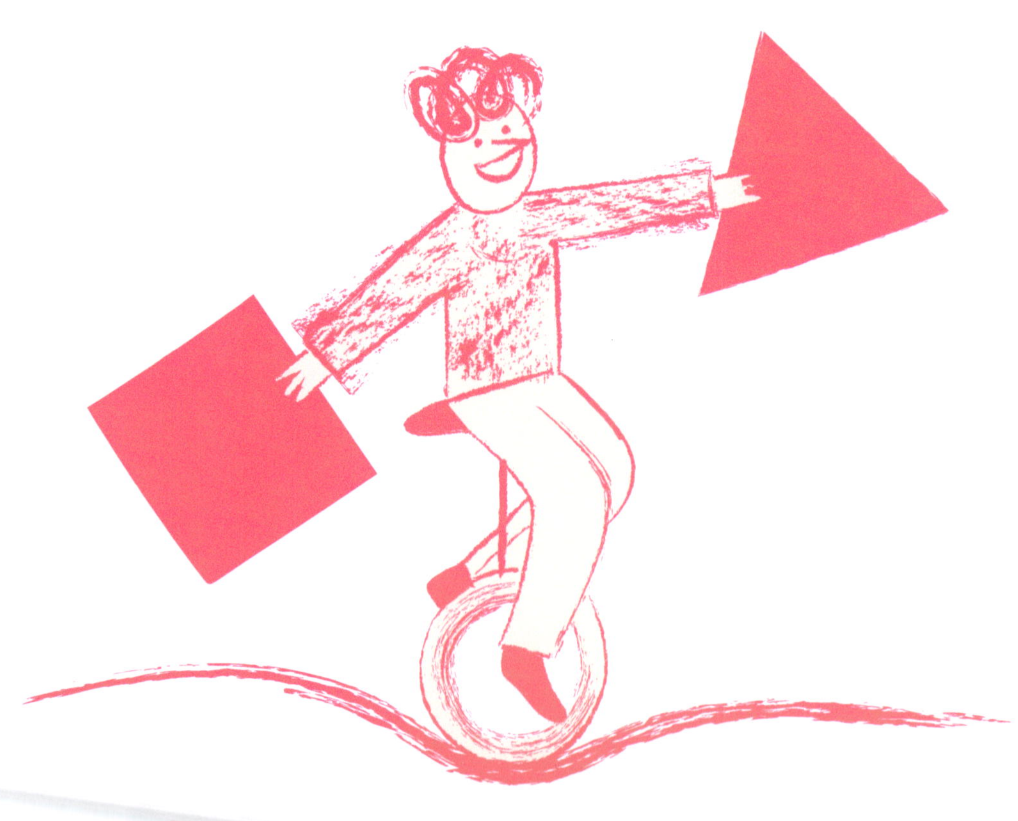

Notes

Notes

Connection & Community

Finding Strength in Others

Day 53

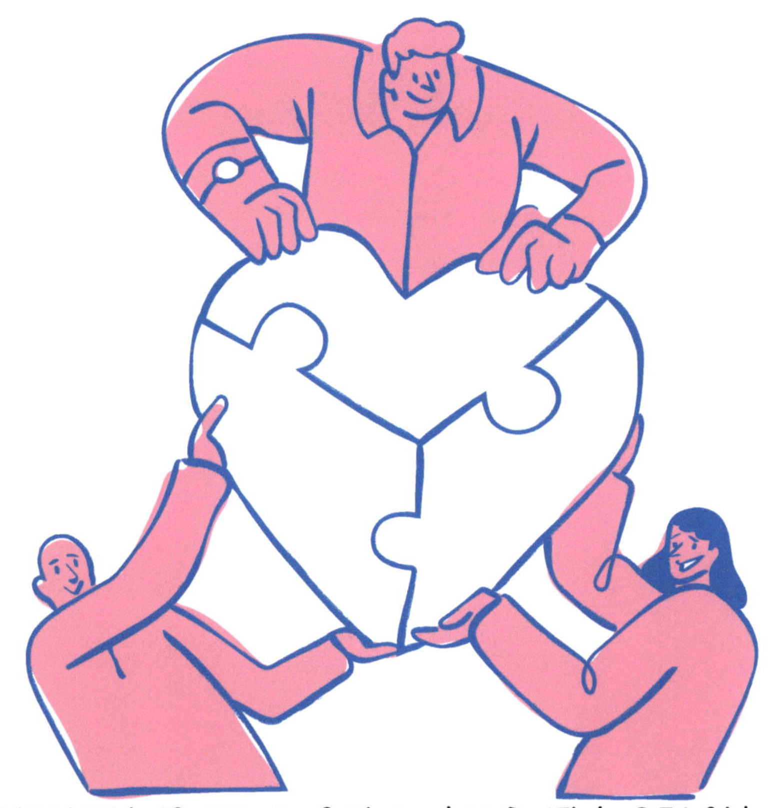

HEALTH ISN'T A SOLO JOURNEY. REACH OUT, CONNECT, AND LET OTHERS INSPIRE YOU.

Day 54

SURROUND YOURSELF WITH PEOPLE WHO SUPPORT YOUR GROWTH. TOGETHER, WE'RE STRONGER.

Day 55

EVERY CONNECTION IS A THREAD IN THE FABRIC OF YOUR WELL-BEING. STRENGTHEN IT WITH KINDNESS AND CARE.

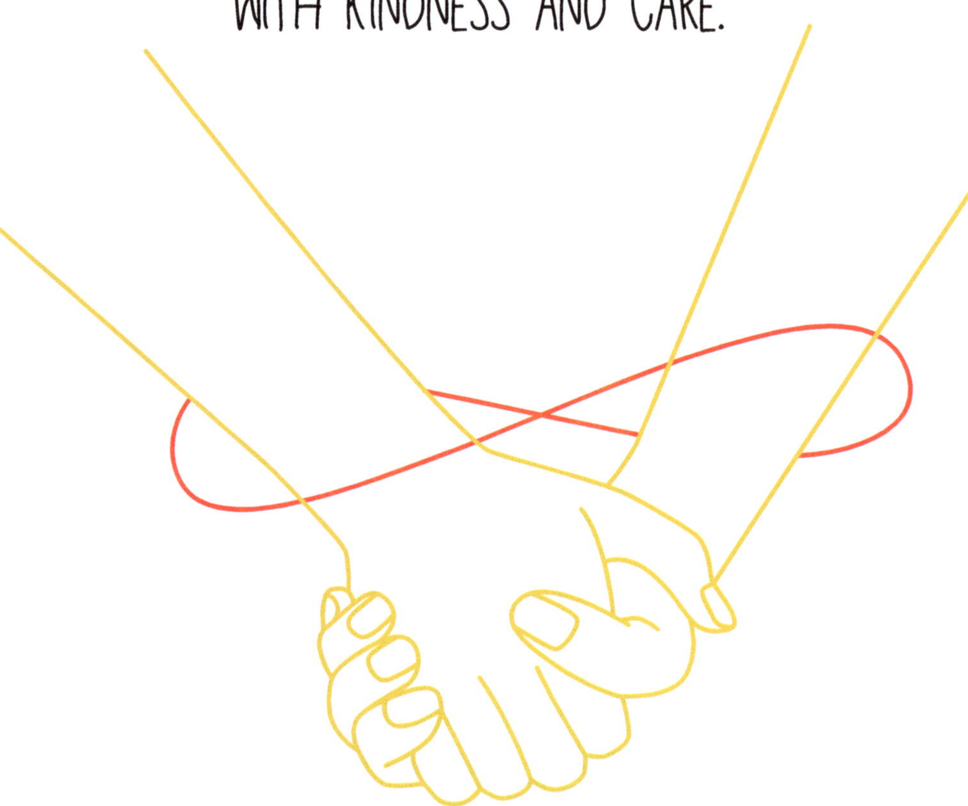

Day 56

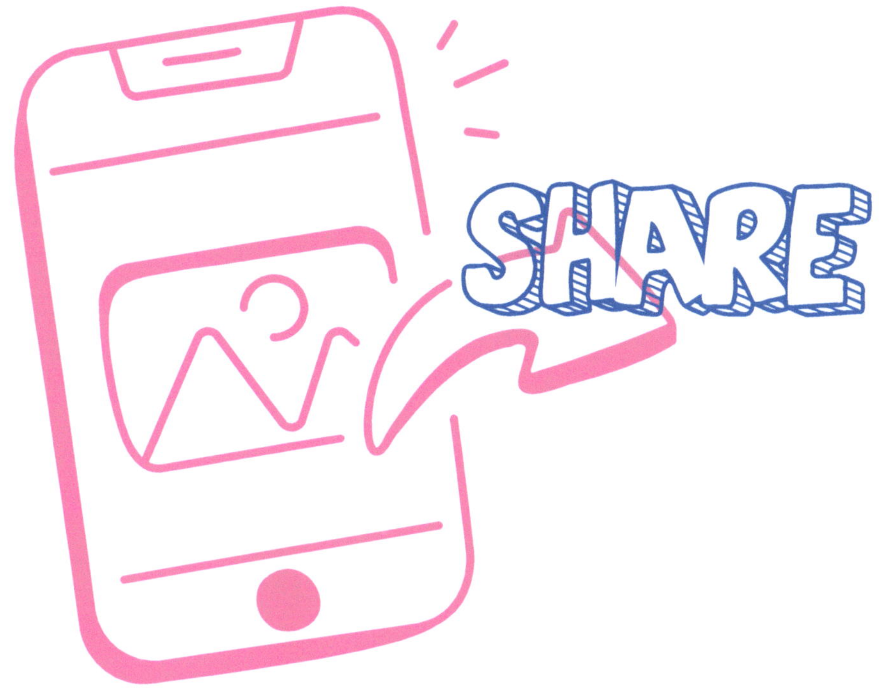

TRUE HEALTH BLOSSOMS WHEN YOU SHARE YOUR JOURNEY WITH OTHERS. LET SUPPORT AND ENCOURAGEMENT FLOW BOTH WAYS.

Day 57

A SIMPLE CONVERSATION CAN BE A POWERFUL REMEDY. OPEN UP, LISTEN, AND LET HEALING HAPPEN IN CONNECTION.

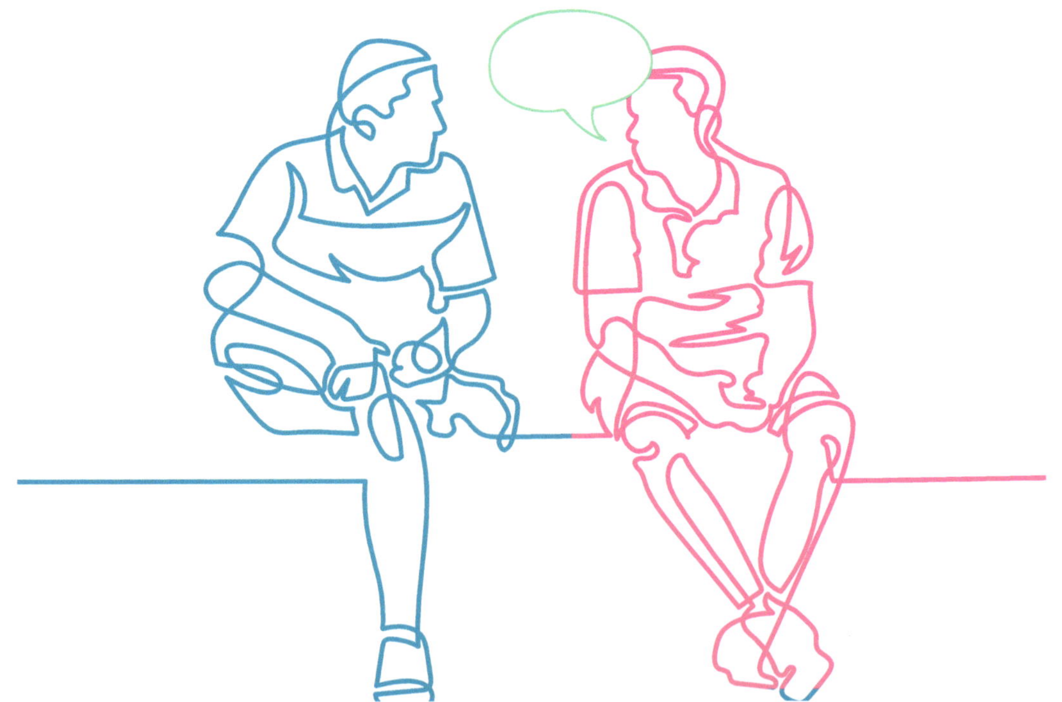

Day 58

LAUGHTER SHARED WITH FRIENDS IS A WORKOUT FOR THE SOUL. SEEK MOMENTS OF JOY IN THE COMPANY OF OTHERS.

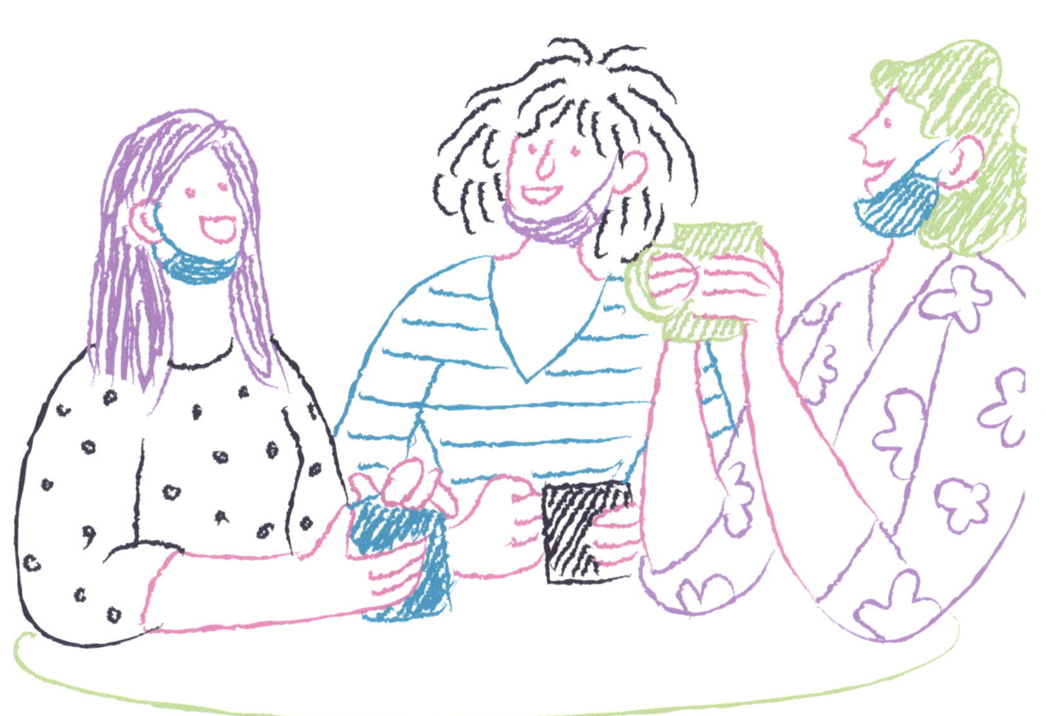

Day 59

LEAN ON SOMEONE WHEN THE LOAD FEELS HEAVY. HEALTH GROWS IN THE BALANCE OF GIVING AND RECEIVING SUPPORT.

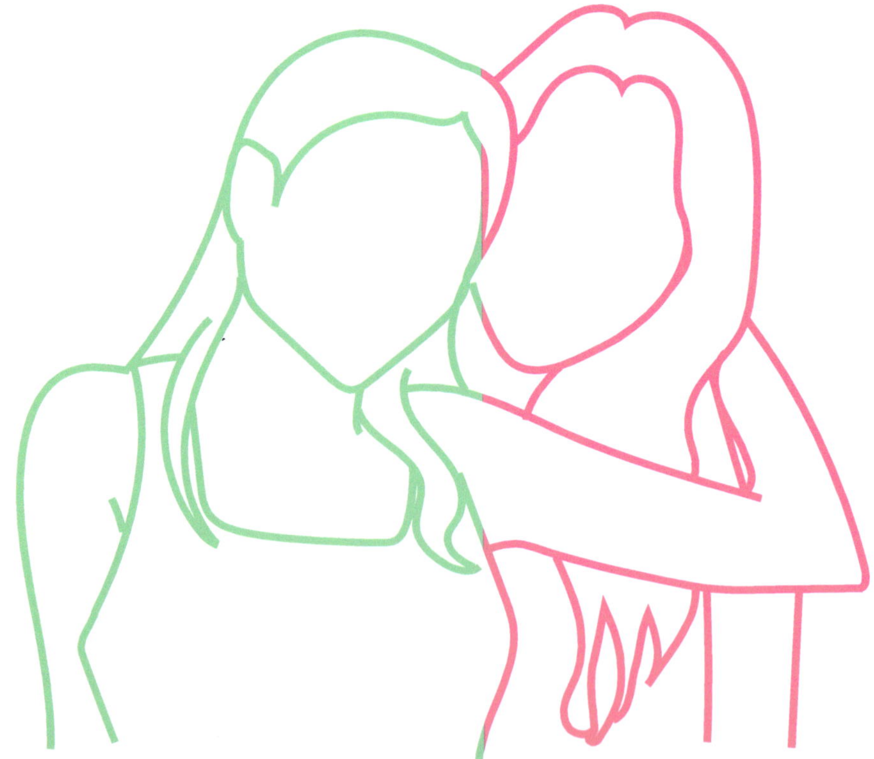

Notes

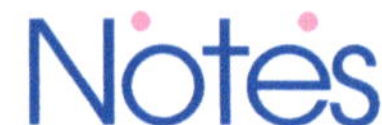

Notes

Embracing Balance

Day 60

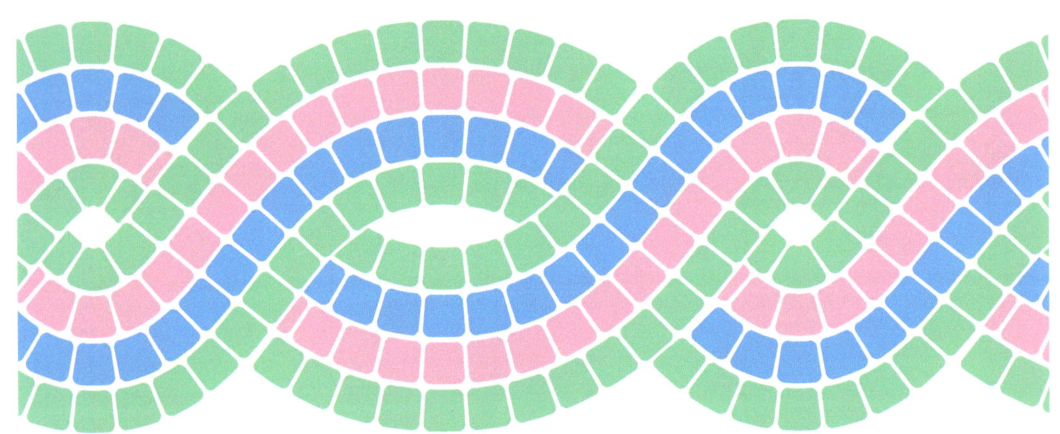

YOUR WELL-BEING IS A MOSAIC. EACH PIECE—
WORK, REST, JOY, AND NOURISHMENT COMES
TOGETHER TO CREATE A BEAUTIFUL WHOLE.

Day 61

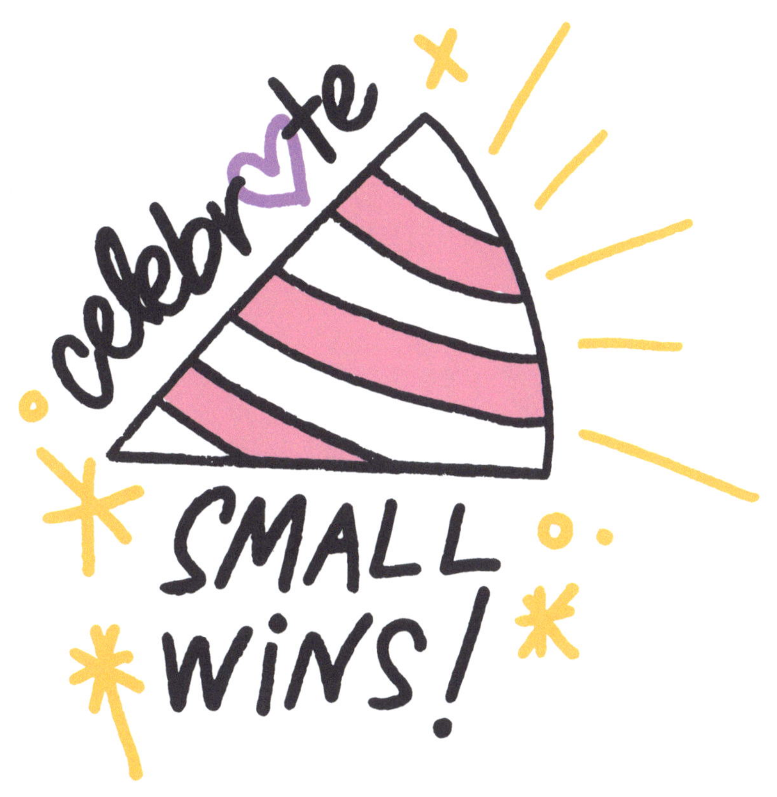

CELEBRATE THE LITTLE WINS. AN EXTRA GLASS OF WATER, A SHORT WALK, OR A MINDFUL MEAL. PROGRESS IS BUILT ON THESE MOMENTS.

Day 62

NOT EVERY DAY WILL BE PERFECT, AND THAT'S OKAY. CONSISTENCY OVER TIME IS WHAT BRINGS REAL CHANGE.

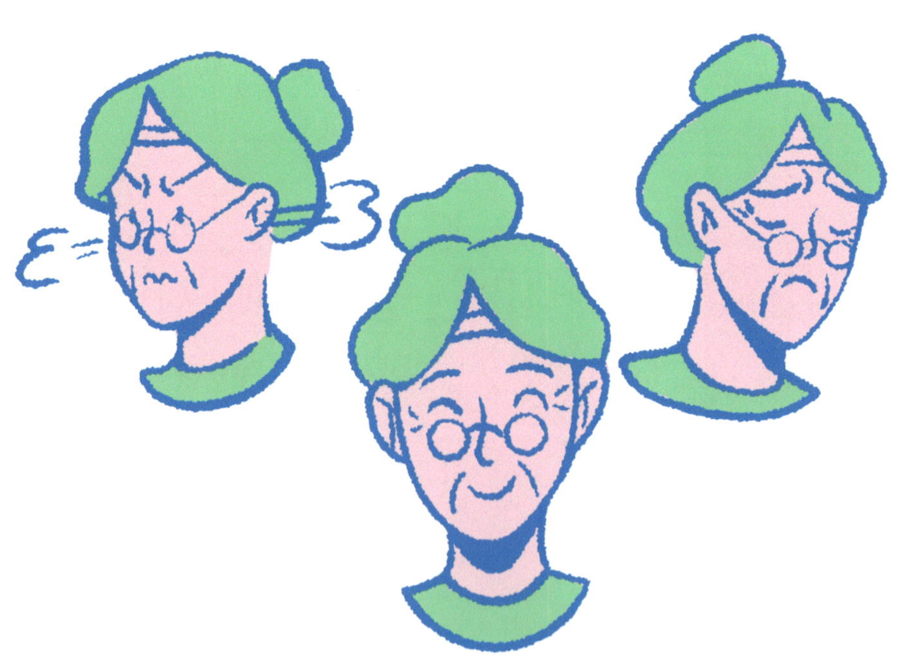

Day 63

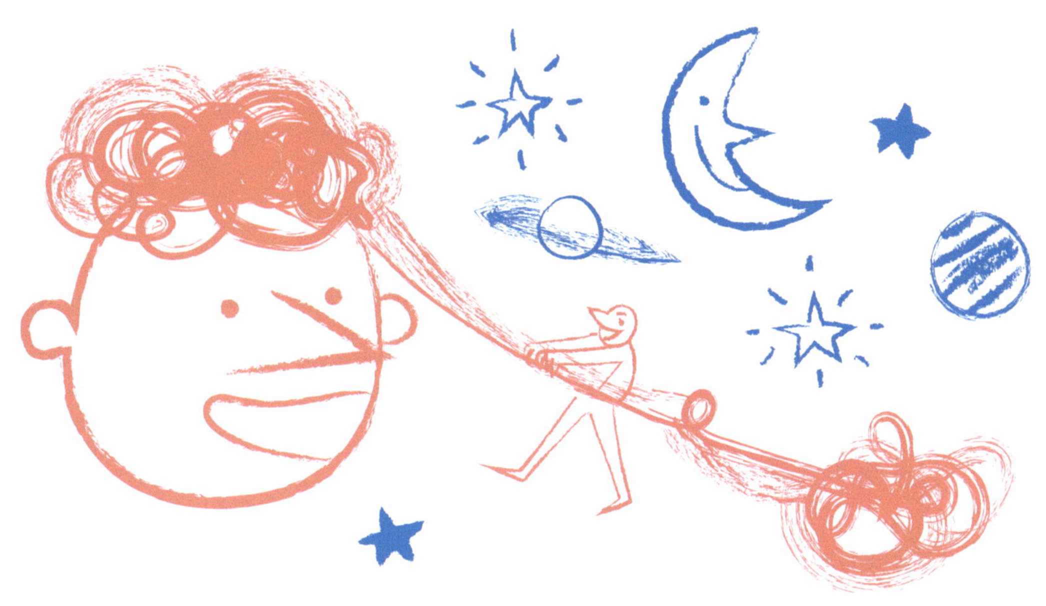

WHEN LIFE FEELS OVERWHELMING, SIMPLIFY. FOCUS ON WHAT NOURISHES YOUR BODY AND CALMS YOUR MIND.

Day 64

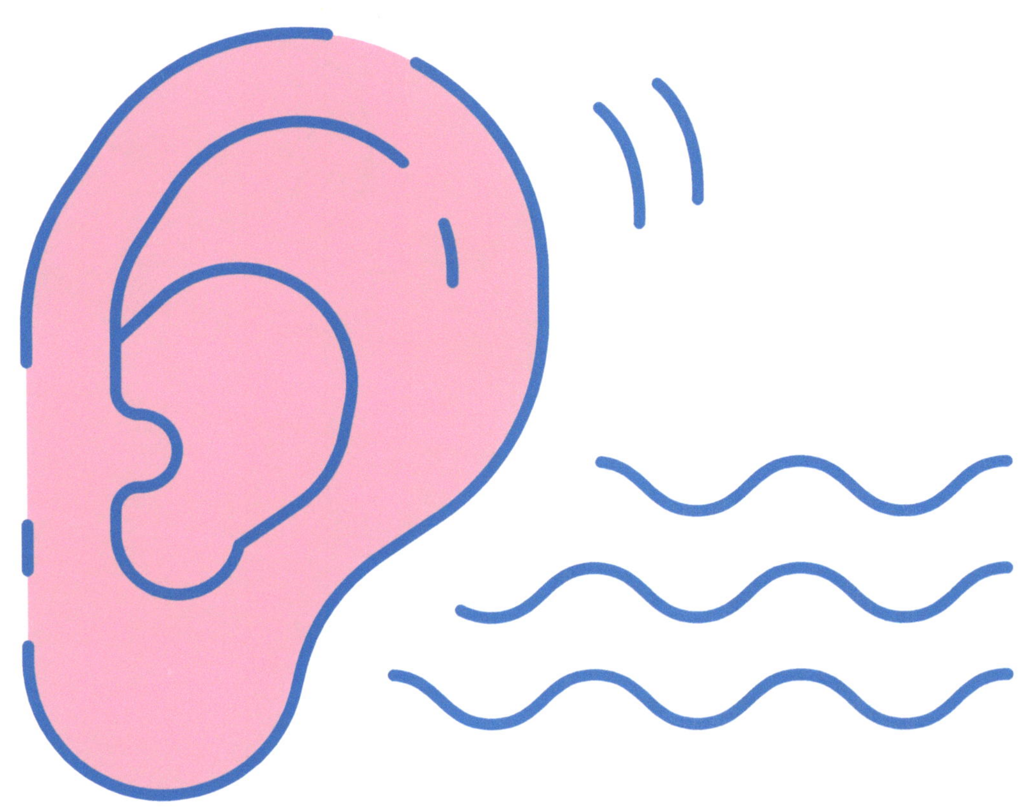

LISTEN TO YOUR BODY'S WHISPERS BEFORE THEY BECOME SHOUTS. BALANCE STARTS WITH TUNING INTO WHAT YOU NEED.

Day 65

TRUE HEALTH IS ABOUT HARMONY, BETWEEN EFFORT AND REST, DISCIPLINE AND INDULGENCE, AND STRIVING AND BEING.

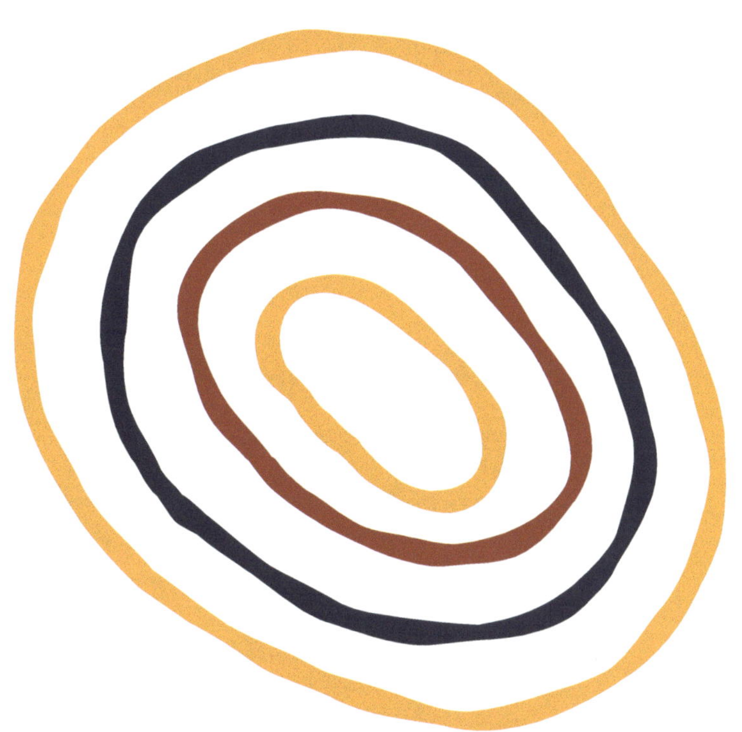

Day 66

BALANCE IS THE ART OF LIVING FULLY, NURTURING YOUR BODY, CALMING YOUR MIND, AND EMBRACING THE MOMENTS IN BETWEEN. IT'S NOT A DESTINATION, BUT THE RHYTHM OF A LIFE WELL-LIVED.

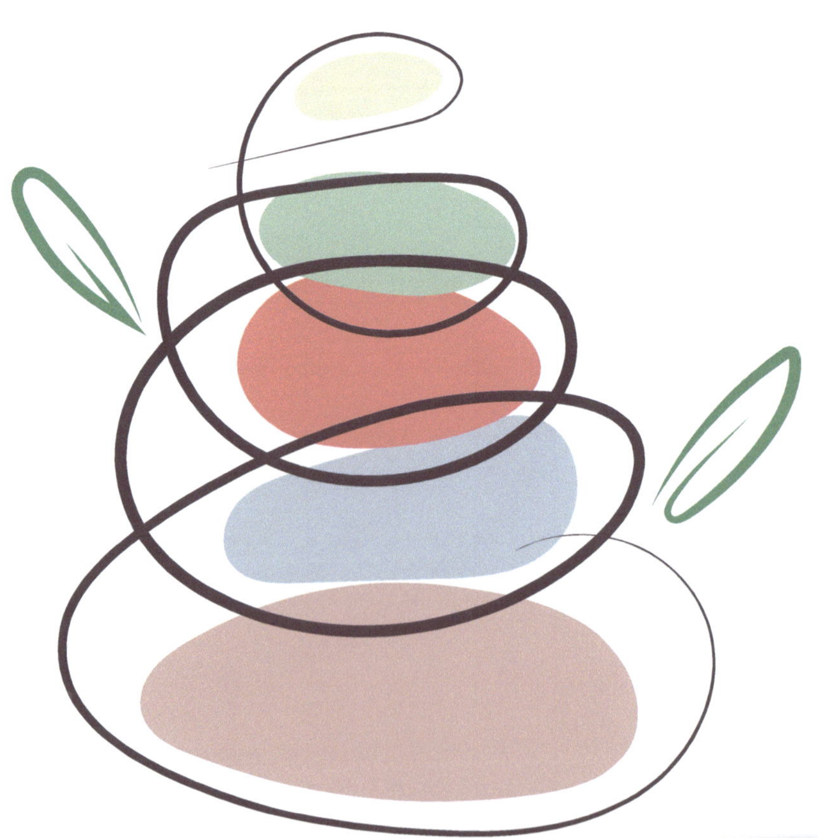

Notes
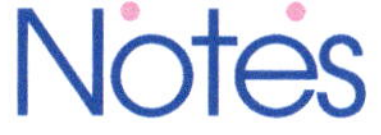

www.ingramcontent.com/pod-product-compliance
Lightning Source LLC
Chambersburg PA
CBHW040902260726
48664CB00025B/1281